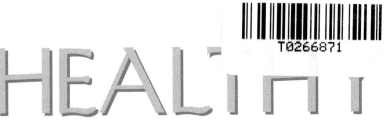

HEALTHY
TRAVEL

HEALTHY TRAVEL

Don't Travel Without It!

Michael P. Zimring, M.D.,
and Lisa Iannucci

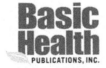

**Basic
Health**
PUBLICATIONS, INC.

The information contained in this book is based upon the research and personal and professional experiences of the authors. It is not intended as a substitute for consulting with your physician or other healthcare provider. Any attempt to diagnose and treat an illness should be done under the direction of a healthcare professional.

The publisher does not advocate the use of any particular healthcare protocol but believes the information in this book should be available to the public. The publisher and authors are not responsible for any adverse effects or consequences resulting from the use of the suggestions, preparations, or procedures discussed in this book. Should the reader have any questions concerning the appropriateness of any procedures or preparation mentioned, the authors and the publisher strongly suggest consulting a professional healthcare advisor.

Basic Health Publications, Inc.
www.basichealthpub.com

Library of Congress Cataloging-in-Publication Data
Zimring, Michael P.

    Healthy travel / Michael P. Zimring, and Lisa Iannucci.
      p. cm.
    Includes bibliographical references and index.
    ISBN 978-1-59120-149-6 (Pbk.)
    ISBN 978-1-68162-732-8 (Hardcover)
   1. Travel—Health aspects. I. Iannucci, Lisa. II. Title.

RA783.5.Z56   2005
613.6'8—dc22   2005012316

Editor: Kate Johnson
Typesetting: Gary A. Rosenberg
Book design: Carol Rosenberg
Cover design: Mike Stromberg

This book is dedicated to my late father, Joseph G. Zimring, M.D.
His love and professional integrity continue to inspire me
to treat my patients with dignity and respect.

—Michael P. Zimring, M.D.

From the time I was young, all I ever wanted in my life was to be a
writer—or so I thought. Then I became a mother and learned that life
is about so much more. This book is dedicated to my three wonderful
children, Nicole, Travis, and Samantha, who made me realize how
good it is to achieve my own dreams and how much better it is to
watch them achieve their own. To the moon, stars, and back, I love
you all so much. And to my mom, Patricia Quaglieri, thanks for
all your never-ending love and support—I love you.

—Lisa Iannucci

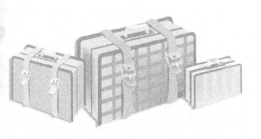

Contents

Acknowledgments

There are several people that I would like to acknowledge for their contributions to the development of this book: Penny, my wife, for supporting me and encouraging me through this new venture; Dr. Walter B. Koppel, my good friend and colleague, for reviewing the manuscript; Dan Collins of Media Relations at Mercy Medical Center, for encouraging me to pursue opportunities that led to this publication; and Lisa Iannucci, my coauthor, for inviting me to collaborate on this project. It was truly a pleasure and educational experience working with Lisa and our editor, Kate Johnson.

—Michael P. Zimring, M.D.

There are several people that I'd like to thank for helping me get this book off the ground: Dr. Michael Zimring for agreeing to take on this project and having great energy and passion for the topic; Dan Collins at Mercy Medical Center in Baltimore for introducing me to Dr. Zimring and encouraging him to work on the project with me; Norman Goldfind for having faith in this book and being one of the most accessible publishers I've ever met; my fellow travel writers and others who shared their personal travel experiences; my talented illustrator Amy Manso; and mostly "Ollie"— my editor Kate Johnson—who kept me on track, does a job well done, and makes this whole process fun.

—Lisa Iannucci

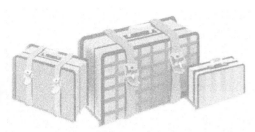

1. A Pre-Trip Checkup

YOU PROBABLY WOULDN'T VENTURE ON A LONG ROAD-TRIP without first giving your car a complete inspection to prevent any potential problems along the highway. You would make sure the tire pressure was correct, the oil was changed, the windshield-wiper fluid was filled, and the roadside emergency kit was stocked.

When you travel, do a similar pre-trip checkup on yourself, your children, and any pets that are going with you. It's important to get medical clearance for travel, especially if you have any preexisting conditions that could flare up or if you have recently undergone surgery. For example, if you have cardiovascular disease, there is nothing wrong with traveling if your condition is stable or compensated. However, you should consult a doctor if you are on medication for acute or chronic cardiovascular disorders. Such factors as intense heat, temperature changes, traveler's diarrhea, and infectious diseases can all place a strain on the circulatory system. This is why it's important to discuss preexisting conditions with your physician ahead of time.

The last thing you need is to be stuck in an airport because you didn't bring the right documents for your medical syringe, stranded in a foreign country without an adequate supply of an essential medication, or in a precarious or even life-threatening position simply because you didn't go to the doctor or dentist before you left home.

APPOINTMENTS, PAPERWORK, AND SUPPLIES

Protecting yourself from any potential medical complications is a matter of education and preparation. Get off to a good start by doing the following as a pre-trip checkup before you leave (for your convenience, a summary of this section is included within the checklists in Chapter 10).

Seek Medical Advice at Least Six Weeks Prior to Departure

You, your spouse, and your children—anyone who will be traveling—should have a medical checkup. This is especially important if you are traveling internationally, if you have any preexisting medical conditions including heart disease, hypertension, or any other chronic condition, or if you have recently had surgery or a heart attack. Schedule appointments with your physicians (and any medical specialists you see regularly) to get medical clearance to travel.

Make a list of your questions before each appointment, bring it with you, and write down the answers so you don't forget anything after you leave the doctor's office. At your checkup, inform the physician of your destination(s), how long you will be away, and how you will be traveling (by car, plane, boat, and the like). Ask about any particular health concerns you may have such as dietary changes, any prescription or over-the-counter medications that you may need, and any suggested or required vaccinations (vaccination details are given later in this chapter). If you are disabled, be sure to discuss all of the medical equipment you might need on your trip.

Visit a Travel Clinic

To prepare properly for the challenges of a journey through "the global village we call earth," travelers should also seek medical advice at a travel clinic at least six weeks prior to departure. Why visit a travel clinic when you already have a personal physician? Because although your physician knows your medical history, he/she may not keep up to date with what's happening all over the country or overseas. To find a travel clinic near you, visit the International Society of Travel Medicine at www.istm.org (click on "Travel Clinic Directory" and put in your search criteria).

The travel physician conducts a risk assessment to determine what health challenges you may face when you're away from home. To do so, he/she takes a personal health history that should include your health problems, medications, allergies, and current immunization status, and then considers several other factors, starting with your destination(s)—and, if there's more than one, the order in which they are to be visited.

Additional factors that determine the degree of risk you will face are the setting of your trip (such as urban, rural, or wilderness) and your style of travel (such as whether you are staying in a first-class hotel, sophisticated resort, local housing, or tent). Whether you are traveling on business, taking the family on a relaxing beach vacation, going mountain climbing, or embarking on a safari or wilderness adventure, the purpose of the trip is an important consideration as well. The physician will also inquire about your "traveler personality." For example, are you content to eat only "safe foods," or are you the type to try anything, such as tempting treats from a street vendor's cart?

Once the assessment is complete, the travel physician will make recommendations including appropriate immunizations, any prophylactic medication(s) you may need, and suggestions for the treatment of minor or annoying illnesses that you may encounter (such as traveler's diarrhea; see Chapter 2).

In addition, a full-service travel clinic can make emergency arrangements so you have someone to call if you develop a serious medical problem or injury while traveling. In conjunction with a travel assistance company (for an example, see the inset on page 5), the travel clinic would be able to coordinate any emergency care with your primary physician, coordinate your care at a foreign destination, and, if necessary, arrange your evacuation for proper care. (See also Chapter 8.)

Research Your Destination

Visit the U.S. Department of State's website at www.state.gov and review the relevant consular information sheet(s). These sheets are available for every country and describe entry requirements, currency regulations, unusual health conditions, crime and security, political disturbances, areas of instability, and special information about driving and road conditions. They also provide addresses and emergency telephone numbers for U.S. embassies and consulates. Find your destination area's embassy and consulate, and record their telephone numbers in your "personal health notebook" (Chapter 10).

Find out about the medical facilities in the area you will be visiting (this is a good idea even if you're only traveling domestically), and check the websites of the Centers for Disease Control and Prevention (www.cdc.gov) and the World Health Organization (www.who.int/ith) to read the most up-to-date health advisories for your destination. You can also find out about medical facilities in your travel area by researching the area's tourism bureaus.

Check Your Medical Insurance Policy and Purchase Additional Coverage

Does your policy cover health care for any illnesses or injuries while you travel? Are you covered if you travel internationally? Are you covered in case of an emergency? In most cases, the answer is no, and you will need traveler's insurance to supplement your existing coverage.

Buy traveler's insurance directly from a medical insurance company (we recommend Medex; see the inset on page 5). Don't buy it from a tour operator! If the operator's business goes under, so does your policy. Make certain that your traveler's insurance is comprehensive and provides coverage regardless of the length of your trip or the activities you decide to enjoy. Your coverage should include everything from physicians' fees, hospital expenses, and dental expenses to the costs of emergency evacuation, repa-

Travel Gaps in Medicare

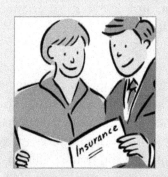

In most cases, Medicare won't pay for health care or supplies outside of the United States. Medicare coverage is also limited when you take a cruise, unless the doctor is allowed (under certain laws) to provide medical services on the cruise ship, and the ship is in a U.S. port or no more than six hours away from a U.S. port when you receive the medical services. However, Medigap—health insurance policies sold by private insurance companies to fill "gaps" in the original Medicare Plan coverage—may offer supplemental coverage for international travel.

To learn more about Medigap before you travel, get a free copy of the *Guide to Health Insurance for People with Medicare: Choosing a Medigap Policy* at the website www.medicare.gov (select "Publications": the guide is CMS Pub. No. 02110) or by calling 800-MEDICARE (800-633-4227, TTY 877-486-2048).

triation arrangements and fees, and transportation for any accompanying travelers. Once you have the insurance, list your policy number and any emergency telephone numbers in your personal health notebook. Give this information to relatives or friends back home as well.

Review Your Medications and Get Proper Paperwork

Bring a sufficient amount of any prescription medications—in their original, labeled bottles—for the entire trip. Carry documents from the prescribing physician that list the physician's name, the name of the medication, the reasons for its use, and other such information (this is especially important for narcotic medication).

If you take prescription narcotics, call the embassy of the country you will be visiting and find out whether you need additional paperwork or forms in order to bring the medication into that country. According to the U.S. Department of State, 2,500 Americans are arrested overseas each year, and a third of these arrests are for drug-related charges. Many people assume that, as United States citizens, they cannot be arrested; but from Asia to Africa and Europe to South America, United States citizens have found out the hard way that drug possession or trafficking equals jail-time in foreign countries. You don't want to be arrested, or detained at the airport, because you don't have the right documents for your medications. "I didn't know it was illegal!" won't get you out of jail.

Ask your doctor or pharmacist whether time changes or high altitudes may change the effectiveness of your medications, and ask about any possible adverse interactions

Worry-free Emergency Coverage: Medex

When researching traveler's insurance, visit the Medex website at www.medexassist.com (or call 800-732-5309 or 800-537-2029). In addition to comprehensive health coverage, Medex can provide assistance twenty-four hours a day, seven days a week, in locating the nearest appropriate care, monitoring your progress, overcoming language barriers, maintaining contact with your primary care physician, and arranging for medical evacuation. Medex also sells medical kits that arm travelers with extra protection that may be needed in the event of the unexpected (see the inset on page 113 in Chapter 8).

Shop for Supplies Before You Travel

Magellan's is a leading "one-stop shop" for travel supplies including first-aid products, clothing care products, jet lag prevention, toiletries, and toilet kits. Check them out online at www.magellans.com while you are planning your trip, or request a free catalog by calling 800-962-4943 or 805-568-5400 (international).

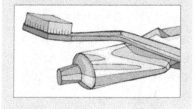

with sun exposure. Know the generic names of your medications, as brand names can vary internationally. Pack any nonprescription medications that you frequently use, like painkillers and antacids, as well as a personal first-aid kit. Remember to keep all necessary medications close at hand at all times.

Once you know what you can and cannot bring, pack a pillbox that has compartments for each day of the week—being away from home and out of your usual routine can make you more likely to forget to take your medication. If you are traveling internationally, don't use the pillbox until you arrive at your destination, and remember to have official labels for any medications, especially narcotics. Meanwhile, keep your medications in their original labeled containers. If you are flying, make sure to pack them in your carry-on bag in case your luggage is lost. If you are traveling by car, have them with you, not in the trunk or in a suitcase.

Visit the Dentist and the Eye Doctor

Whether or not you're in a strange city, you definitely don't need a toothache. Having a dental checkup beforehand can reduce your chances of a toothache or gum problem on the road. If you wear eyeglasses or contact lenses but don't have an extra pair, consider buying them for the trip in case something happens to your primary pair. Also, the dry air on airplanes can cause dry eyes, so you may want to consider leaving your contact lenses at home and simply traveling with glasses.

Take Pets to the Vet

If Paws and Claws will be traveling with you, make sure they are healthy enough to travel and have enough of any necessary medication for the duration of your trip. Carry documents from the veterinarian that list the

Online Records and Reminders

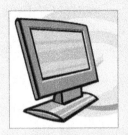

What if you have a medical emergency while traveling, and healthcare personnel need your medical history? Before you leave, visit your "personal MD" at the website www.personalmd.com. Created by Executive Health Exams International, the site helps you organize health records for yourself and your family. These records, which are accessible "24/7," can include basic information and emergency contacts, current health conditions, allergies, drug sensitivities, family history, personal history, immunizations, and information on medical devices.

Changing daily schedules and even time zones can cause chaos when you're trying to remember when to take your medication (or give yourself a shot; see Diabetes and Other "Syringe Travel" on page 11). If you need a reminder, RemindRx at www.personalmd.com can take care of it. The service also reminds subscribers to go to doctors' appointments, take birth control pills, and the like. Reminders can be sent to your pager, cell phone, personal digital assistant (PDA), and/or email account.

prescribing vet's name and contact information, the name of the medication (brand names can vary, so know the generic name as well), the reasons for its use, and so forth, in case of any emergency.

If you are traveling to a tick-infested area, discuss with your vet whether your pet needs a Lyme vaccination. According to the website www.camp-a-roo.com, it's also important to see whether your dog needs other special medications such as that for heartworm. This determination is made, through a simple test, for dogs older than six months. Heartworm medication is recommended for dogs going along the Pacific Coast north of Monterey, into the Sierras, and to Texas, the Midwest, or the eastern coastal states. For dogs living in California's San Marcos Pass or other areas where heartworm is common, the site also says, "Giardia vaccination should be given if you'll be hiking in the local mountains, or in areas that are swampy or are associated with stagnant water or creek beds (in the Santa Barbara area, this includes East Beach, the UCSB [University of California at Santa Barbara] slough, and Lake Los Carneros)."

If you are traveling internationally, be aware that certain countries require pets to be quarantined for up to six months before they are allowed entry. At the very least, you will need to take a written statement of your pet's health from the vet to confirm that your pet is disease-free and up to date on vaccines, including a rabies vaccination at least thirty days in advance.

SPECIAL NEEDS

Some travelers have to consider special health circumstances like pregnancy, diabetes (or any other syringe-related condition), and physical disabilities. It's important to understand how these conditions may be affected during your travel, and what precautions you can take to prevent any complications. Remember that most countries, especially third-world countries, are not like the United States in requiring special accommodations for people with physical challenges.

Moms-to-Be

Less than a decade ago, a pregnant woman got the okay from her doctor when she wanted to fly, as long as she was healthy and her pregnancy was normal. Today, we really do not want to advise all pregnant women to refrain from traveling, but all the risks of travel must be weighed against the benefits.

Any pregnant would-be traveler should consult her obstetrician, in conjunction with a travel physician, to correlate all the relative contraindications of travel to a given area, so that an educated decision regarding travel can be made. Obviously, it's unwise for a pregnant woman to visit a country endemic for such diseases as malaria or yellow fever (see Vaccinations on page 17). In general, it is considered unwise to travel in the third trimester, and most airlines won't accept a passenger in her last month of pregnancy.

Cosmic radiation in the atmosphere at high altitudes has always been a concern for moms-to-be, but that's really not anything to worry about, according to Iffath Hoskins, M.D., chair of the Department of Obstetrics and Gynecology at New York University Downtown Hospital: "If you're only taking one flight, the radiation isn't enough to cause absolute harm, although it's more than the woman would get if she was on the ground."

Hoskins says, however, that the air on a plane isn't clean, and that a pregnant woman's suppressed immune system is susceptible to airborne infections and illnesses. She adds, "Also, a developing fetus needs high amounts of oxygen, and air on a plane has a decreased oxygen pressure, so you're not breathing in as much oxygen."

Pregnant passengers who sit too long in the same position are also at a higher risk for the blood clots known as deep vein thrombosis or DVT (see Chapter 3). The extra estrogen in a pregnant woman's system adversely impacts her body's ability to prevent blood clots. If a long flight cannot be avoided, physical movement is the best DVT prevention.

In-flight Care

American Airlines (www.AA.com) has introduced the SkycAAre Program to provide skilled medical companions for travelers who need limited medical attention or care during their flight. All medical companions on American Airlines flights are registered nurses, usually flight nurses.

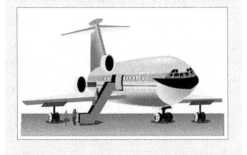

If you absolutely must fly, Hoskins recommends booking your flight for the middle third (months four, five, and six) of your pregnancy: "The first trimester has the higher risk of miscarriage and the last trimester has the highest risk of preterm labor, but the middle third is considered a safe zone, where there is no risk for structural damage and you're the most comfortable."

In the absence of federal or international airline regulations concerning pregnant passengers, each airline has its own rules, but most require a note from the obstetrician if a passenger is thirty-six or more weeks pregnant. Can you deliver on the plane? Although it's a rare occurrence, it has happened. There are currently no regulations, however, that require airlines to carry obstetrical equipment.

If you decide to travel abroad while pregnant, quality medical care is important for you and your unborn baby, so research your destination as mentioned earlier. "If you are going to Spain, for example, you have to know the standard of medical care," says Hoskins. "A five-hour bus ride will take that long to get back to getting care. You also have to understand the medications and treatment and see if it's similar to what you would get in the United States."

Here are some additional tips for traveling moms-to-be:

- See your obstetrician or midwife before you leave, and get a complete checkup as close to your departure as possible. Again, make sure you have documentation from your obstetrician that clears you for travel, as well as documentation for any prescriptions.

- Check your health insurance—and your travel insurance policy, if you have one—for coverage of pregnancy-related conditions including delivery and neonatal care.

- Know the nearest hospital (and the quality of care provided) at your destination. Don't just rely on knowing a specific doctor in the area, because there is a good chance that a particular doctor may not be on call that night.

- When you're pregnant, don't try to save money by taking flights with layovers. If possible, take a one-leg flight instead of a connection.

- Don't travel back and forth on the same day. Stay overnight to give yourself time to rest and to stretch your legs.

- Drink plenty of bottled water—and in third-world countries, bottled carbonated water is even safer (discarded water bottles can be refilled with local tap water and resold, but this is harder to do with carbonated water).

- Maintain your mobility on the plane or train: get up, move around, and circle your ankles to increase blood flow. If you are traveling by car, stop at least every two hours and get out for no less than fifteen minutes.

- Pack enough snacks to maintain your energy level and avoid low blood sugar.

- Use the pillows on a plane flight, and ask for a seat with more legroom if available. Put the seatbelt under your belly and over your hips, not across the middle of your belly.

- If you are going out of the country, consult your doctor about vaccination requirements.

- Avoid high-altitude destinations, where oxygen to the fetus could be decreased.

- Visit your airline's website to review its particular requirements for pregnant passengers. For example, American Airlines (www.AA.com) lists the following: "In addition to the information below, please also be aware that a medical certificate is required if you will be traveling within four weeks of your delivery date in a normal, uncomplicated pregnancy . . . For domestic flights under five hours [not including travel over water], travel is not permitted within seven days before and after your delivery date. If you should need to travel within seven days before or after delivery, a medical certificate is required as well as clearance from our Special Assistance Coordinator . . . For international travel or any flights over the water, travel is not advised within thirty days of the due date, unless you are examined by an obstetrician within forty-eight hours of outbound departure and certified in writing as medically stable for flight. Travel within ten days of the due date for international travel must have clearance from our Special Assistance Coordinator. Travel within seven days after delivery requires clearance as well."

Diabetes and Other "Syringe Travel"

Traveling with syringes for patients with diabetes or other diseases caused concern and confusion among airline passengers after September 11th. To help clear the air, we've listed below (with permission) the most recent information from the U.S. Transportation Security Administration (TSA) for individuals traveling within the fifty states who have syringe-related medical conditions. This information only applies to travel within the United States and is subject to change. If you're traveling internationally, consult your airline for applicable international regulations. Check the TSA website at www.tsa.gov for the most up-to-date information before you leave.

- Notify the security screener that you have diabetes or another medical condition such as hepatitis and are carrying your supplies with you. Make sure you have a letter from your physician stating your condition, the medication that you use, and any other pertinent information.

- Make sure a professionally printed pharmaceutical label identifying the medication accompanies your insulin vials, insulin pens, jet injectors, and pump. Since the prescription label is usually on the outside of the box containing the insulin vials or pens, it is recommended that passengers refrain from discarding their insulin box and come prepared with their insulin in its original pharmaceutically labeled box.

- There is no limitation on the number of empty syringes that may be carried through the security checkpoint. Insulin must be with you, however, in order to carry syringes through the checkpoint.

- Lancets, blood glucose meters, and blood glucose test strips can be carried through the security checkpoint.

- For passengers who test their blood glucose levels but who do not require insulin, boarding with lancets is acceptable as long as the lancets are capped and are brought aboard with a glucose meter that has the manufacturer's name embossed on it (as in a One Touch meter imprinted "One Touch Ultra").

- If you are wearing an insulin pump, notify the screeners and request that they visually inspect the pump rather than removing it from your body.

- Advise screeners when you are experiencing low blood glucose and are in need of medical assistance.

The TSA also states, "Should a passenger with diabetes be denied boarding a flight or be faced with any other unforeseen diabetes-related difficulty while passing through security checkpoints, he or she should speak with the security checkpoint supervisor. If the problem is not resolved to the passenger's satisfaction or if a passenger feels he or she has been discriminated against or treated unfairly by federal security checkpoint personnel, please contact the TSA hotline at 1-866-289-9673."

The American Diabetes Association (ADA) suggests that diabetic patients "pack at least twice the number of supplies needed during travel, and bring a quick-acting source of glucose to treat low blood glucose, as well as an easy-to-carry snack such as a nutrition bar. Carry or wear medical identification and carry contact information for your physician while traveling. It may also be helpful to have contact information for a healthcare professional available at your destination, and be prepared to adjust medication when traveling in different time zones." The ADA also monitors the security requirements of diabetic airline passengers and can keep you informed of new developments. Check the ADA's website at www.diabetes.org, and call 703-549-1500 extension 1768 to report any difficulties you encounter when you are traveling.

Note: Diabetic travelers who are crossing time zones will need to adjust the timing and dosage of their insulin shots, and should consult a travel physician for an individualized plan to address this situation.

Disabled Travelers

The Department of Transportation (DOT) has issued guidelines regarding the treatment of disabled passengers, their devices, and their assistants. According to the guidelines, individuals assisting passengers with disabilities are still allowed beyond the screener checkpoints at airports. These individuals may be required to present themselves at the airline's check-in desk and receive a pass allowing them to go through the screener checkpoint without a ticket. The guidelines also state that bags for medical supplies and assistive devices are still allowed, once they have successfully passed the security checkpoint too. (See the inset on page 14.)

To ease the frustration of airport logistics and to protect your devices, request any carts or other service you may require when you make your reservation. Describe your limitations and needs, let your travel agent or airline know if you have a wheelchair or guide dog, and ask about the size of the plane and the bathroom.

Simplify security checks by removing any removable parts of your device, if possible, as you will know how to reassemble them. Stay with

"Step Aside, Please": Are You Radioactive?

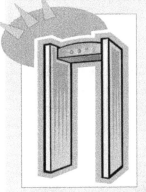

Radiation detectors are now being used in various parts of the country to help fight the threat of terrorism. Most people are not aware that the small amounts of radioactive substances used in certain medical procedures can set off these detectors, and that detectable levels of radiation can still be present in the body for several hours to several months later. Among the most noteworthy of these procedures are iodine isotope therapy for thyroid cancer or hyperthyroidism (overactive thyroid), thallium stress tests of cardiac function, and brachytherapy (implantation of radioactive "seeds") for prostate cancer. Even patients who have simply had a thyroid or bone scan may set off radiation alarms for several days afterward. Therefore, if you have had any type of testing or treatment involving radioactivity, you should carry a note from your physician when you travel.

The DOT Fact Sheet
for Disabled Passengers

This Fact Sheet provides information about the accessibility requirements in air travel in light of strengthened security measures by providing a few examples of the types of accommodations and services that
must be provided to passengers with disabilities. The examples listed
below are not all-inclusive and are simply meant to provide answers to
frequently asked questions since September 11th concerning the air
travels of people with disabilities.

Check-in

- Air carriers must provide meet and assist service (e.g., assistance to
gate or aircraft) at drop-off points. The lack of curbside check-in, for certain airlines at some airports, has not changed the requirement for meet-
and-assist service at drop-off points.

Screener Checkpoints

- Ticketed passengers with their own oxygen for use on the ground
are allowed beyond the screener checkpoints with their oxygen canisters
once the canisters have been thoroughly inspected. If there is a request
for oxygen at the gate for a qualified passenger with a disability, commercial oxygen providers are allowed beyond the screener checkpoints
with oxygen canisters once the canisters have been thoroughly inspected. Commercial oxygen providers may be required to present themselves at the airline's check-in desk and receive a "pass" allowing them to
go through the screener checkpoint without a ticket.

- The limit of one carry-on bag and one personal bag (e.g., purse or
briefcase) for each traveler does not apply to medical supplies and/or
assistive devices. Passengers with disabilities generally may carry medical equipment, medications, and assistive devices on board the aircraft.

- All persons allowed beyond the screener checkpoints may be
searched. This will usually be done through the use of a handheld metal
detector, whenever possible. Passengers may also be patted down during security screenings, and this is even more likely if the passenger

uses a wheelchair and is unable to stand up. Private screenings remain an option for persons in wheelchairs.

- Service animals, once inspected to ensure prohibited items are not concealed, are permitted on board an aircraft. Any backpack or side-pack that is carried on the animal will be manually inspected or put through the X-ray machines. The service animal's halter may be removed for inspection.

- Assistive devices, such as walking canes, once inspected to ensure prohibited items are not concealed, are permitted on board an aircraft. Assistive devices such as augmentative communication devices and Braille 'n Speaks will go through the same sort of security screening processes as used for personal computers.

- Syringes are permitted on board once it is determined that the person has a documented medical need for the syringe.

- Personal wheelchairs and battery-powered scooters may still be used to reach departure gates after they are inspected to ensure that they do not present a security risk. Any backpack or side-pack that is carried on the wheelchair will be manually inspected or put through the X-ray machines.

- Personal wheelchairs will still be allowed to be stowed on board an aircraft.

- Air carriers must ensure that qualified individuals with a disability, including those with vision or hearing impairments, have timely access to information, such as new security measures, the carriers provide to other passengers. For example, on flights to Reagan Washington National Airport, persons are verbally warned to use the restrooms more than half an hour before arrival since after that point in time passengers are required to remain in their seats. Alternative formats are necessary to ensure that all passengers, especially deaf persons, understand new security measures such as the one at Reagan Washington National.

Reprinted courtesy of the Office of the Assistant General Counsel for Aviation Enforcement and Proceedings and its Aviation Consumer Protection Division, issued on 10/29/01.

the device during the checks so you can answer any questions that security personnel may have about it. In addition, keep any paperwork handy that describes your medical condition and the need for your items. This is especially helpful for the security personnel if you cannot communicate well, and it might prevent potential misunderstandings about your device.

Visit these two websites about traveling with a disability: www.flying-with-disability.org and www.makoa.org. These sites also include information on organizations that offer package tours and cruises for those with special needs.

Travel Tips for People with Hearing Loss

For people with hearing loss or deafness, traveling can sometimes entail a unique set of frustrations. Any traveler who is deaf or hard of hearing should, of course, always carry a notepad and pen or pencil to communicate in writing whenever necessary. Experts at the National Technical Institute for the Deaf in Rochester, New York also recommend taking the opportunity to educate people about communication and to avail yourself of the various communication technologies at your disposal, as follows:

- When flying, be sure to tell the flight attendant at the gate and on the plane that you have a hearing loss, so he/she can inform you of any announcements.

- If you have wireless Internet access, you can use it *en route* to check your flight's status at the airline's website, as well as to make, change, or cancel any travel reservations (flight, lodging, or car rental) and to obtain directions.

- You can also call the airline, hotel, or car-rental company through a wireless relay service.

- When you make your hotel reservation, inquire about the availability of an American Disabilities Act (ADA) kit. Offered at many hotels, an ADA-accessible kit includes such items as a teletypewriter or TTY (also called a telecommunication display device or TDD, which allows both parties who have one to type messages directly to each other via a phone line), a door strobe, and a fire alarm. If your hotel doesn't have a TTY or an ADA-accessible kit, suggest that the manager call a neighboring hotel to borrow one for the duration of your stay.

- Inform the hotel staff that you are deaf or hard of hearing, so they'll know to check your room in case of an emergency or evacuation. They can also be helpful in giving you phone messages, calling for take-out, and the like.

- For safety reasons, however, be sure that the staff keeps your hearing loss in confidence. Once, for example, when a sign was posted on a hotel room door that the guest was deaf, her room was broken into while she was sleeping.

VACCINATIONS

Everyone, including children, should be up to date on the usual childhood vaccinations before embarking on worldwide exploration. Some diseases that have been essentially eradicated in the United States can still be acquired elsewhere. Measles, for example, has recently broken out in Mexico, the Congo, and the Marshall Islands, and Panama now requires proof of measles vaccination for travelers from other South American countries. Vaccinations are not the norm in many third-world or developing countries, where lower standards of health care and hygiene increase the health risk of the traveler who takes our higher standards for granted.

Be aware of your immunization status in regard to tetanus, diphtheria, hepatitis, measles, rubella, mumps, and varicella. Older adults should be up to date on influenza and pneumonia vaccinations if indicated. Influenza and pneumonia vaccinations are also important if you tend to become exhausted or poorly hydrated when traveling, especially if you will be in crowds or confined to enclosed spaces with other people who might be harboring communicable diseases (for example, during airplane, train, or bus travel, or on cruises).

Let's take a look at several frequently given vaccinations and their importance. You should discuss the pros and cons of each with your travel physician. (*Note:* In addition to the following, we could discuss vaccinations for other diseases including plague, tick-borne encephalitis, and tuberculosis, but most of these vaccines are unavailable or of limited availability in the United States, and are only needed by people traveling under very special circumstances.)

Tetanus and Diphtheria

These two vaccinations are usually given together. Tetanus, also known as lockjaw, is a neurological disorder caused by contamination of a wound (such as a skin puncture, burn, or surgical incision) by certain bacteria found in the soil or in feces. The disorder leads to increased muscle tone and generalized spasms, and can be deadly. Tetanus is found throughout the world, but is fully preventable by proper vaccination. Whether you travel or not, you should update your tetanus immunization at least every ten years.

Diphtheria is an acute bacterial disease that causes respiratory obstruction and/or skin lesions. The bacteria's toxin can also affect the heart, kidneys, and nerves. Diphtheria is transmitted by respiratory droplets or by close contact with someone who already has the disease. Diphtheria remains a problem in countries where vaccination is not available, such as in the former Soviet Union and parts of Eastern Europe.

Hepatitis

Anyone traveling outside of the United States should be vaccinated against hepatitis A and B. Hepatitis A is a highly contagious viral disease that can be transmitted from person to person, or spread through the fecal-oral route by ingestion of water or food (like shellfish) contaminated with the feces of someone who has the disease, especially in areas of poor sanitary conditions such as developing countries. In children, a case of hepatitis A may be mild, but in adults it may be severe. One shot is good for approximately two years, and getting a booster shot will keep you immune for ten or more years.

Hepatitis B is a viral disease that is usually transmitted via the parenteral route (that is, intravenously, intramuscularly, or subcutaneously) by body fluids such as blood, through intimate personal or sexual contact (as well as from pregnant mother to fetus). If a motor vehicle accident—the major cause of morbidity or mortality for travelers—lands you at a healthcare facility in a developing country, your risk of contracting hepatitis B through transfusions of blood or plasma products is high. Sterility of medical instruments in such facilities is also questionable, and non-sterile instruments are another source of hepatitis B transmission. The risk of contracting the disease is elevated if you spend time with the local population in underdeveloped countries where hepatitis B is endemic (widespread).

All newborns in the United States are now vaccinated against hepatitis B. In some parts of the country, childhood vaccination for hepatitis A is also routinely provided, depending on the incidence of the disease in that area. Getting a hepatitis B vaccination might be a good idea for adults who missed this opportunity as a child, though it might not be a high priority for a short tourist trip. This vaccination is typically given as three shots over a six-month period, but an accelerated schedule is also quite effective. It would probably be wise to get the Twinrix A/B (GlaxoSmithKline) vaccination, which might be more convenient for people who require or desire protection against both hepatitis A and B, as it entails fewer shots and is more efficient in the long run.

Typhoid Fever

Typhoid fever is a systemic bacterial disease that can cause prolonged fever, abdominal pain, intestinal bleeding, delirium, and coma. Like hepatitis A, it is contracted through the oral-fecal route in developing countries, from food or water that is contaminated as a result of poor sewage treatment and/or water treatment. Typhoid fever vaccine can be administered orally or as a shot.

Caution: If you are currently taking a proton pump inhibitor such as Prilosec, Prevacid, Protonix, Nexium, Aciphex, or similar drugs, you are more susceptible to contracting typhoid from contaminated food or water, because these drugs reduce the stomach's gastric acid barrier, allowing even a small inoculum (dose of bacteria) to cause infection. (This is also the case for traveler's diarrhea; see Chapter 2.)

Polio

Polio, also called infantile paralysis, is a disease that destroys parts of the nervous system and can cause paralysis of the muscles controlling such vital functions as breathing. It is still found in some underdeveloped countries where hygiene standards are poor and people live in crowded conditions. Even if an adult traveler received a polio vaccination series in childhood, he/she should be immunized again with the parenteral or the intramuscular injection as opposed to the oral vaccine. This adult polio booster should then be good for life.

Yellow Fever

Yellow fever is an acute, mosquito-borne, viral infection that can be quite serious, causing liver failure as well as affecting other vital organs such as the kidney and heart. The fatality rate is over 20 percent.

Yellow fever is the only vaccination that is required by the World Health Organization. Certain governments in the "yellow fever belt" of South America and Africa require travelers to get this vaccination ten days prior to entering the country. Other governments simply recommend it in general (and it would be wise to follow that recommendation), but might require it if you are coming from another country where yellow fever is found, whether or not you spent time in specifically endemic areas.

The vaccine contains a live virus and has several important contraindications that you should discuss with your travel physician. The injection must be administered by a Certified Yellow Fever Vaccination Center, which will issue a special Yellow Card with a certification stamp. A booster shot is required every ten years to fulfill the immunization requirements.

Meningococcal Meningitis

Outbreaks of meningococcal meningitis, a devastating bacterial disease that is spread through respiratory droplets or person-to-person contact, typically occur among people living in close quarters (military barracks, for example). The disease is especially associated with epidemics in crowded conditions such as the massive Hajj pilgrimage in Saudi Arabia. The vaccine is usually given to travelers who will be visiting the "meningitis belt" in sub-Saharan Africa and spending time with the local population. Some universities require a meningococcal meningitis vaccination for students who will be living in dorms, and the Saudi Arabian government also requires this vaccination for pilgrims to the Hajj.

Rabies

Rabies is a devastating viral disease that is usually fatal. Adventure travelers or other travelers who are likely to come in contact with animals are at the greatest risk of contracting rabies: these include hikers and bikers, as well as tourists or business travelers who venture out for an early morning jog in endemic areas. Most municipalities in the United States require rabies vaccinations for domestic animals, but you shouldn't count on this requirement in developing countries.

If you are bitten or scratched by a rabies-infected animal, it's important to seek proper treatment even if that means evacuation to an appropriate facility. Fortunately, there is a pre-exposure rabies vaccination, and having it will make the post-exposure treatment less complicated.

Japanese Encephalitis

Japanese encephalitis is caused by a mosquito-borne virus that affects the central nervous system. The transmission cycle of this virus involves mosquitoes and farm animals such as pigs. Found in parts of Southeast Asia, Japanese encephalitis usually occurs in rural farming areas but can also occur in suburban areas of large cities.

To determine whether or not you should be vaccinated against this disease, your travel physician should consider the duration of your stay in an endemic area and the frequency of your involvement in significant outdoor activities. Because of the delayed hypersensitivity reactions—even as serious as anaphylaxis (a life-threatening allergic response)—that are associated with the vaccine, its risk/benefit ratio must be thoroughly assessed.

POST-TRIP CHECKUP

Even if you do not experience any medical complications or illnesses while traveling—and let's hope you don't—make sure to visit your travel physician when you return, especially if you:

- Spent three or more months in a rural area of a developing country

- Were told that you have (or think that you may have) malaria

- Were treated or hospitalized for any medical illness

- Continue to have any symptoms or develop any unexplained symptoms

- Or, are simply unsure whether any of your activities increased your risk of exposure to certain conditions or diseases

If you have persistent diarrhea, especially with mucus or blood, or have an unexplained fever, you should seek medical advice. (See Chapter 2 for information about traveler's diarrhea.) If you traveled through a malarial area and have an unexplained fever, you are considered to have malaria until it is proven otherwise, even if you followed the proper precautions (including taking prophylactic antimalarial pills and using mosquito repellants and insecticides). Remember, it only takes one bite from one infected mosquito. In addition, if you miss a dose or two of the malaria medication, or if you get a considerable amount of mosquito bites, your chances of contracting malaria are increased.

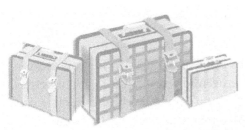

2. Prepare to Stay Healthy

YOU'VE WAITED A LONG TIME FOR THIS TRIP, your work is done, you scheduled your vacation time, the tickets are purchased, and you're almost on your way. The last thing on your mind is getting sick. Unfortunately, getting sick happens, and it can definitely throw a wrench into your plans or even sideline you for a few days or weeks.

When traveling, even the healthiest body is subjected to a host of possible infections and diseases. In Chapter 1, we presented the immunizations that will help protect you from some of those conditions. There are, however, some illnesses for which there are no vaccinations.

You can catch a cold, flu, or gastrointestinal virus virtually anywhere. If you eat food that has not been properly prepared, you may end up with traveler's diarrhea. A trip to the mountains may sound like fun, but if you travel too high too fast you could suffer from high-altitude sickness. And that annoying bug bite could end up giving you Lyme disease or malaria. (Two other extremely important health issues for travelers, deep vein thrombosis and jet lag, are covered in Chapter 3.)

This book is intended to make you a *smart and healthy* traveler, which means being aware of possible complications. Yes, you can encounter myriad conditions and diseases while traveling; the point of this chapter is not to panic you, but to thoroughly prepare you. You will see, however, that we're not going to go into great detail about every disease or illness because, honestly, all the health risks in every part of the world are too much to cover in a book of this size and scope.

Instead, we want this book to be a catalyst for you. Although it's fun to just book a trip and take off on an adventure, it's important to protect your health. When you're done reading this book and are ready for your next journey, we want you to get on the Internet and research the region where you will be traveling, learn about that region's potential health risks, and most of all, make sure you are fully prepared to travel (see the Resources section at the back of the book). The more informed you are, the healthier you'll be and the more fun you'll have.

Don't Dry Out

To counteract nasal dryness on the plane, dab a little gel such as Vaseline around your nostrils. Try Aquaphor Healing Ointment to moisturize chapped lips and dry skin patches; it can also serve as a skin protector on the faces of adults and babies in bitter cold and winds. This ointment is available at drugstores or online at www.drugstore.com and www.Aqua phorHealing.com.

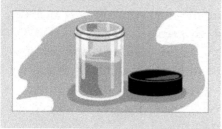

FLYING THE HEALTHY SKIES

Can flying actually make you sick? On her sixteen-hour flight to New Zealand, travel writer Arline Zatz was dizzy and feverish and had crushing ear pain. Margaret Littman, another travel writer and editor, gets a sinus infection every time she flies. (*Author's note: I painfully remember my first flight . . . I boarded the plane feeling fine and anticipating my visit with an old college friend; the next day, I came down with a horrific cold that put a damper on my entire vacation. —Lisa*) Coincidence? Maybe. But studies have shown that flying poses an increased risk of contracting influenza, bronchitis, tuberculosis, and more.

THE AIR UP THERE

There is an increased chance of bacterial or viral transmission in a confined, crowded environment like an airplane, and the longer your flight, the more at risk you are for inhaling germ-contaminated air. Cabin air is dry, with only 5 to 20 percent humidity; such low humidity makes respiratory conditions worse, and the resulting dehydration can also be a contributing factor to the development of a deep vein thrombus (see Chapter 3). In addition, cabin air pressure is usually pressurized to 8,000 feet, which causes problems for some people, especially those with chronic lung disease.

Keep in mind that several other factors increase your risk of contracting an illness when you fly. For example, if you are like many travelers who are busy preparing for a journey, you probably won't sleep well the night before. You'll be checking last-minute details, getting the house in order, or just feeling too excited about your trip. You may also assume that you'll catch up on your sleep on the plane—after all, it's a vacation and you're going to kick back and take it easy, right?

Washed Up?

Wash your hands frequently throughout your trip to reduce your chances of contamination!

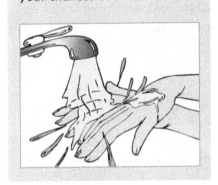

However, if you're not well rested and well hydrated, you are already starting your excursion on a bad note. Already you have lowered your immune system's defenses, leaving you susceptible to catching a cold or other virus. Add to this any health conditions, medication side effects, the consumption of alcohol, and even motion sickness; couple these with the fact that you're in a small area with hundreds of other sniffling and sneezing passengers who are touching the same handrails, doorknobs, and trays; and your chances of infection increase dramatically.

According to the U.S. Food and Drug Administration (FDA), what you're at risk for is exposure to more than 200 different viruses known to cause symptoms of the common cold. Some viruses, such as the rhinoviruses, seldom produce serious illnesses. Others, such as parainfluenza and respiratory syncytial virus, produce mild infections. Common cold symptoms may include runny nose, sore throat, sneezing, and body aches, and usually appear two to three days after the virus enters your body.

(Author's note: Remember my cold from my first flight? When I thought about it, I realized that I hadn't slept well the few nights before because I was nervous and excited. I had also been running myself ragged getting errands done for the trip. Plus, it was the beginning of January—cold season—so before I even left, all the factors were already in place for me to catch a cold on the trip. —Lisa)

The Ol' One-two Punch: Health Products to Pack

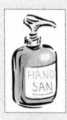 **Hand sanitizer.** Of course a hand sanitizer doesn't take the place of a good lather of soap and water, but it can't hurt to keep a bottle of the stuff in your carry-on bag in case normal hand-washing is temporarily impossible. Purell (www.purell.com) makes an instant, alcohol-based hand sanitizer that kills most of the common germs that cause illness.

 Echinacea. The herb *Echinacea purpurea* has been said to boost the immune system by stimulating the body's production of infection-fighting white blood cells. Start taking it five days before you leave for vacation, take it during your trip, and continue taking it five days after your return.

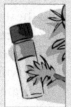 **Homeopathic cold remedies.** For many of us, it's an expression of Murphy's Law: plan a trip, get a cold. Flying with a cold can be downright painful, but not everyone wants to load up on medications that can produce drowsiness. Zicam (www.zicam.com) claims its over-the-counter homeopathic cold remedies (nasal gel pump, nasal swabs, chewable or rapid-melt tablets, and oral mist) reduce the duration of cold symptoms without making you tired. Colds can take a week or more to go away on their own, but travelers can't afford to be sick for that long, and Zicam may help.

Caution: Be careful about combining medications and/or herbal products.

But what if you are already saddled with a head cold before you travel? Should you postpone your flight? It all depends on whether you have sinus congestion or ear pain. Changes in plane cabin air pressure have been known to disturb a normal ear and cause pain. The American Academy of Family Physicians (AAFP) states that such a pressure change may result in trauma to an ear that is already compromised. So, if your sinuses and the eustachian tubes in your ears are already swollen from a cold, changes in cabin air pressure can make the pressure in both much worse. According to the AAFP, this can adversely affect the middle ear, leading to pain and possibly a ruptured eardrum with bleeding.

"Keep Out da Noise, Keep Out da Pop!"

Changes in cabin pressure can cause painful popping in the ears, especially for children. Chew gum and also have your child chew gum to restore the balance of pressure during takeoff and especially during landing. For younger children, bottle-feeding during this time can be helpful. Eardrops are also available to ease the pain, but consult your physician before using them.

It is recommended that you ground yourself when you are not feeling well, whether it's a cold, sinus infection, or flu, and wait to fly until you feel better. If you must travel, ask your physician about over-the-counter medicine for your symptoms. You may want to take a medication for sinus congestion or aches and pains, but some drugs can cause drowsiness, impaired judgment and vision, upset stomach or bowels, or even itching. Taking a decongestant, which is recommended to help reduce regular ear pain when flying, may also cause stimulation, so be sure not to combine a decongestant with caffeine.

Want to save your ears from airplane noise? Try Plane Quiet Active Noise Canceling Headphones (www.protravelgear.com). This product won the "Best of the Best" and "Best Technology" awards from *Travel Insider,* a widely read weekly Internet publication. The soft, ergonomic headset lowers 17 decibels across the sound spectrum, so you can relax and enjoy your favorite movie, music, or soothing silence on your next flight or anytime you need to block out unpleasant noise. The headset is compact, weighs less than 6 ounces, and folds to fit easily into your carry-on bag. A single AA battery provides a minimum of fourteen hours of continuous use. Plane Quiet is compatible with all airline in-flight entertainment systems and portable electronic devices.

LEPTO . . . WHAT?

You've probably heard of traveler's diarrhea, but what about leptospirosis? Is SARS still a concern for travelers? Do you think that only chickens get avian flu? It's important to know about such illnesses, from the mundane to the exotic.

SARS and Avian Flu

Severe acute respiratory syndrome or SARS is a new viral illness that begins with a high fever. Further symptoms can include headache, body aches, mild respiratory symptoms, diarrhea, and a dry cough. After several days, the illness may lead to pneumonia. It's important to be aware, especially if you are traveling to or from a SARS-affected area, that symptoms of this syndrome mimic the flu. The symptoms can appear within ten days after infection. Before your trip, check the CDC's website (www.cdc.gov) for any travel restrictions related to SARS. Be sure to take precautions (good hygiene!) when traveling, and notify your physician immediately if you show signs of the syndrome.

Avian influenza or "bird flu," which is spread through poultry and other birds, has also been found in humans in such Asian countries as Thailand, Cambodia, Laos, and Vietnam, where it is thought to have been transmitted directly from infected poultry or from their excretions or droppings. This disease can be easily confused with typical flu symptoms like fever, chills, sweats, and muscle aches and pains. Avian flu, however, is more severe, with a high fatality rate. Some of the drugs presently used to treat viral diseases have no effect on avian flu. At press time, a vaccine is being tested.

Advice to travelers from the CDC at press time is to avoid contact with live-animal markets and poultry farms in those countries affected by avian flu. Recent reports also discuss the possibility of "gene swapping" between avian and human influenza viruses when a person is infected with both, which could possibly lead to human-to-human transmission of the newly mutated flu subtype. For this reason, it's still important to get your regular influenza vaccination. Again, check the CDC's website before you travel for the most updated information on avian flu.

Leptospirosis

If you enjoy swimming, kayaking, white-water rafting, biking, or hunting, you (and any animal traveling with you) may be at risk for exposure to the spirochete organism *Leptospira interrogans*. Leptospirosis, a disease associated with wild and domesticated animals, is spread mainly through the urine of infected animals. Some outbreaks of leptospirosis have occurred in the United States, the Caribbean, South America, and Malaysia, and infection can also occur in urban and household settings elsewhere in the world. Symptoms include fever, headache, and conjunctivitis. The infection can lead to kidney dysfunction, jaundice, hemorrhage, and aseptic meningitis. Fortunately, a wide variety of antibiotics including doxycycline and penicillin are effective treatment for the disease. As for prevention, the avoidance of swimming in contaminated freshwater or walking barefoot on moist contaminated soil would be a good start. Prophylactic (preventive) doxycycline is also useful for travelers to areas endemic for both leptospirosis and malaria.

Schistosomiasis

Schistosomiasis, also known as bilharziasis, is caused by the parasitic worms *Schistosoma mansoni, S. haematobium,* or *S. japonicum,* collectively called schistosomes. Although schistosomiasis is not found in the United States, 200 million people are infected worldwide annually. Infection can occur when your skin comes in contact with freshwater in which certain types of snails that carry schistosomes are living. Within days after infection, you may develop a rash or itchy skin, and fever, chills, cough, and muscle aches can begin within one to two months of infection; many people, however, have no symptoms in these early phases of the disease. Safe and effective drugs, taken in pill form for one to two days, are available for the treatment of schistosomiasis.

Traveler's Diarrhea

According to the CDC, each year 20 to 50 percent of international travelers are affected by traveler's diarrhea or TD. All you have to do to get TD is to eat food or drink water that is contaminated with *Escherichia coli* bacteria, commonly known as *E. coli.* Symptoms include increased volume and frequency of bowel movements, watery bowel movements, cramping, bloating, fever, and general malaise. TD can last from a few days to a few weeks—and it can absolutely ruin a vacation.

High-risk areas for getting TD are Mexico, Central and South America, Africa, the Middle East, Asia, or any developing or third-world country. You are also at high risk if you are a young adult; if you have an immunosuppressed medical condition, inflammatory bowel disease, or diabetes; or if you take an H2 blocker (such as Zantac or Pepcid), a proton pump inhibitor (such as Nexium or Prilosec), or antacids, because these drugs lower the acid barrier of the gastrointestinal tract, allowing even a small amount of bacteria to cause an infection.

To prevent TD, do not eat raw or undercooked meat and seafood; do not eat raw fruits or vegetables (unless you have peeled them); avoid drinking water that hasn't been boiled or isn't in sealed bottles (this means ice cubes, too, and see the note about water in Chapter 1); and—as enticing as it may be—avoid eating or drinking anything purchased from a street vendor. These precautions are especially important in areas that seem to be unclean.

If you do come down with TD, you can take an antiperistolic agent like Imodium A-D to slow the movement of material through the digestive tract, thereby controlling the diarrhea. A better treatment for TD is a prescription antibiotic such as Bactrim, Vibramycin, Cipro, Noroxin, or Levoquin. Each drug has pros and cons, and some are contraindicated for children or pregnancy, so you and a doctor must determine which choice is best for you. Imodium can be used in combination with these antibiotics. Antiperistolic agents (including Imodium) should NOT be used, however, if you have an invasive diarrhea as evidenced by blood or mucus, severe abdominal pain or bloating, or a fever.

According to a study conducted by the manufacturers of Imodium, 73 percent of Americans report not carrying medication for diarrhea while traveling, and yet more than one in five surveyed ranked diarrhea as the health condition they fear most while traveling. Pack Imodium A-D! *Caution:* Be quite cautious of taking bismuth subsalicylate, more commonly known by the brand names Pepto-Bismol and Bismed, as it has many possible interactions with other medications and medical conditions (see the inset below).

The National Institutes of Health (NIH, www.nih.gov) advises that you do not take bismuth subsalicylate if you are taking any of the following medications:

- Anticoagulants (blood thinners)

- Heparin (the combination of salicylates may increase the chance of bleeding)

- Antidiabetics, oral (diabetes medicine taken by mouth: the combination may bring the blood sugar level too low)

- Medicine for pain and/or inflammation, except narcotics (if the

Pepto Is a No-No

Do not use bismuth subsalicylate if you've ever had any unusual or allergic reaction to it or to other subsalicylates such as aspirin or methyl salicylate (oil of wintergreen), or to other similar medications, including ibuprofen. Do not use it if you are pregnant. If you have dysentery, gout, hemophilia, kidney disease, or a stomach ulcer, check with a doctor before taking it. Do not give bismuth subsalicylate to children under three years of age.

analgesic or anti-inflammatory contains salicylates, the combination of salicylates may lead to increased side effects or overdose)

- Probenecid, also called Benemid, or sulfinpyrazone, also called Anturane (bismuth subsalicylate may make these medicines less effective for treating gout)

- Tetracycline, oral (medicine taken by mouth for infection; the tablet form of bismuth subsalicylate should be taken at least one to three hours before or after tetracycline, or it may decrease the tetracycline's effectiveness)

The most serious complication of TD is dehydration. To replenish fluids, drink plenty of clear liquids and then eat only bland foods. Avoid foods and beverages that could make the diarrhea worse, such as fruits, vegetables, fried or spicy foods, bran, candy, and caffeine. One of the most important things you can do for dehydration is increase your fluid intake.

TD is rarely life threatening for the average, healthy individual, but it can be serious if you become severely dehydrated, so watch for warning signs of dizziness and lightheadedness, dry mouth, increased thirst, decreased urination, and wrinkled skin. If TD symptoms continue even though you have tried treatment, get evaluated by a hospital, physician, or travel clinic to rule out a possible parasitic infection.

Some travelers would like to take a preventive medication to ward off TD on their trip, but this is usually not recommended, unless (1) your trip is very short and you cannot afford to miss one day of pleasure or work, or (2) you are taking an H2 blocker or proton pump inhibitor (see the earlier note about this on page 29), or (3) you are immunocompromised with a disease like Crohn's disease, cancer, or HIV disease. We recommend discussing these or other personal circumstances with your travel physician.

Another form of TD—at times much more serious—is cholera. Cholera doesn't usually affect the average traveler and is an uncommon illness because the organism responsible is typically found in remote places with poor sanitation; however, if you are traveling to remote places or perhaps doing missionary work, you may be at an increased risk of contracting it. Your risk of getting cholera is also higher if you travel to Latin America, Africa, Asia, or the Indian subcontinent.

Cholera is an intestinal infection caused by consuming water or food (for example, raw shellfish; see Chapter 7) that is contaminated with the

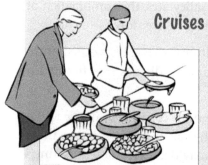

Cruises and Tummy Bugs

When passengers on cruise ships get queasy, it's most likely seasickness, but when hundreds of passengers get diarrhea, vomiting, and stomach cramps, it's time to worry. In 2002, a gastrointestinal virus known as the Norwalk virus spread through many major cruise lines and panicked cruise lovers. But in fact, such outbreaks are infrequent, and the cruise industry is doing everything it can to keep ships clean and passengers healthy.

The CDC suggests doing your homework before booking a cruise. Check out the CDC website's Green Sheet (www.cdc.gov/nceh/vsp/scores/legend.htm) to make sure your intended ship meets sanitation standards. This doesn't guarantee that there won't be an outbreak, but you'll be doing your best to minimize your risk. Once again, hand-washing is a key component to preventing infection with such viruses (remember to bring your hand sanitizer!). Make sure you are up to date on your tetanus, diphtheria, and hepatitis A shots, too (see Chapter 1).

bacterium *Vibrio cholerae*. It is not spread from person to person. Symptoms include profuse watery diarrhea, vomiting, and leg cramps. Cholera causes a rapid loss of body fluids, leading to severe dehydration and shock; without treatment, death can occur within hours. Cholera vaccine is no longer available in the United States (and when it was available, it wasn't very effective), but the illness can be treated with antibiotics and by promptly replacing the fluid loss with an oral rehydration solution. Severe cases may require intravenous fluid replacement.

Motion Sickness

The NIH (www.nih.gov) defines motion sickness as dizziness, sweating, nausea, vomiting, and generalized discomfort experienced when an individual is in motion. Travelers can suffer from airsickness, seasickness, or carsickness. Although it is unpleasant and annoying and can put a crick in your plans, motion sickness is not usually incapacitating.

Academy of Otolaryngology (AAO; www.
ce is maintained by a complex interaction
us system:

yrinth), which monitor the directions of
forward-backward, side-to-side, and up-and-

which monitor where the body is in space (upside down, right
side up, and so on) and also directions of motion.

- The skin pressure receptors such as in the joints and spine, which tell what part of the body is down and touching the ground.

- The muscle and joint sensory receptors, which tell what parts of the body are moving.

- The central nervous system (the brain and spinal cord), which processes all the bits of information from the four other systems to make some coordinated sense out of it all."

Motion sickness occurs when parts of this system are out of sync with each other. For example, the AAO explains that when your airplane is going through patches of turbulence, "Your eyes do not detect all this motion because all you see is the inside of the airplane. Then your brain receives messages that do not match with each other. You might become 'air sick.'"

The AAO suggests the following several methods for preventing and treating motion sickness:

1. Always ride where your eyes will see the same motion that your body and inner ears feel. That is, sit in the front seat of the car and look at the distant scenery; go up on the deck of the ship and watch the horizon; sit by the window of the airplane and look outside. In an airplane, choose a seat over the wings where the motion is the least.

2. Do not read while traveling if you are subject to motion sickness, and do not sit in a seat facing backward.

3. Do not watch or talk to another traveler who is having motion sickness.

4. Avoid strong odors and spicy or greasy foods immediately before and during your travel.

5. Medical research has not yet investigated the effectiven[...]
   folk remedies, such as soda crackers and Seven Up or col[...]
   ice. Take one of the varieties of motion sickness medicines b[...]
   travel begins, as recommended by your physician."

Some medications for motion sickness (such as Dramamine, Bon[...]
Marezine, and others) can be purchased without a prescription, but y[...]
should discuss dosage with your physician. Stronger medicines such as
tranquilizers and nervous system depressants will require a prescription.
Another possibility, also available by prescription only, is scopolamine
absorbed through the skin from a small medicated patch (Transderm
Scop) worn behind the ear. The patch should be applied at least four hours
before traveling and changed every three days.

You can also try the following remedies:

- Pressure-point bracelets that apply pressure to a specific point on the
  wrist, which is supposed to suppress nausea and vomiting.

- Ginger root (*Zingiber officinalis*), fresh or in various other forms: "You
  can drink fresh ginger tea, eat slices of candied ginger, or take the pow-
  dered spice in capsules . . . if you do not like its strong flavor," says Dr.
  Andrew Weil on his website, www.drweil.com. "Try ginger immediately
  before you travel if you are susceptible to this malady [motion sickness],
  or eat it at the first sign of discomfort."

Acute Mountain Sickness

Nancy Monson wishes she could forget her first flight to Aspen, Colorado
from New York. After landing, she had a headache and trouble breathing,
vomited, and felt sluggish. "I thought I had the flu," says Nancy. "I rested
for a day, didn't do very much, drank lots of water, avoided alcohol, and
got a good night's sleep. I felt much better the next day."

But it wasn't the flu that was laboring Nancy's breathing. A doctor diagnosed her with a mild form of acute mountain sickness, which is caused by
a lack of oxygen in thin mountain air that results in less oxygen in your
lungs. The higher you go, the greater the effects. Symptoms like Nancy's
usually appear within the first forty-eight hours. If you continue to ascend
while suffering from warning signs, or if the symptoms are left untreated,
your condition can get worse and you may even die.

Studies have shown that rapid decompression of an airplane's cabin can also cause mild symptoms of altitude sickness. With planes flying higher than ever before, it is becoming increasingly important for travelers to be aware of the symptoms and treatment of this condition. Acute mountain sickness is a particular concern for air travelers who depart from a location at sea level and arrive within hours at altitudes of 8,000–13,000 feet without adequate time for the body to adjust.

If you find you're short of breath, confused, or can't walk in a tandem, then descend and sleep at a lower level, because symptoms can worsen while you sleep. The best way to prevent any form of mountain illness is to ascend slowly and give your body time to adjust.

Another danger at the heights traveled by skiers and mountain-climbers is a condition called high-altitude pulmonary edema, or HAPE. HAPE is a life-threatening form of fluid in the lungs that can occur in otherwise healthy people. Most symptoms appear at elevations greater than 8,000 feet. The classic HAPE sufferer is young and well conditioned, and there is a slightly greater incidence in men than in women.

Diamox is quite useful for prevention or treatment of mountain illness. You can acclimate faster to a high altitude by taking 125 milligrams of Diamox twice a day starting one or two days before your ascent and continuing to take it for two to three more days after your arrival at the desired altitude. Diamox, however, is a sulfa drug that should not be used by anyone who is allergic to sulfa, and its side effects include abnormal skin sensations, extra thirst, and some effect on taste. Other drugs used to prevent or treat altitude-related illness are Decadron, Adalat, and Procardia. Anyone traveling to high altitudes should consult a travel physician about the appropriateness of any of these medications. *Reminder:* If you will be traveling to high altitudes for mountain climbing, a ski trip, or any other reason, tell your doctor beforehand.

Here are a few more tips on combating mountain illness:

- Avoid alcohol, sleeping pills, and narcotics.

- Do not overdo activities the first day. Limit your first twenty-four to thirty-six hours to adjusting to your new environment. After that, you can participate in more activities.

- Remember that your heart is working harder than usual. Do not exert yourself any more than necessary.

- Drink more water than usual.

● If you are currently on medications, high altitudes may change their effectiveness, so be sure to check with your doctor about this ahead of time.

Bug Bites

"Creepy-crawlies" from mosquitoes, bees, and fleas to spiders, biting flies, and ticks can wreak havoc on your body and your trip. Like Mother said (okay, it was Benjamin Franklin, but Mom too), an ounce of prevention is worth a pound of cure, so be prepared! What types of critters can you expect to, ahem . . . bug you? It depends on where you travel, but outdoorsman Brian Brawdy (www.brianbrawdy.com) cautions travelers to be most concerned with ticks and mosquitoes.

Ticks

Ticks are small insects that bite (painlessly), fasten themselves onto skin, and feed on blood. Found in tall grass and shrubby vegetation, ticks can also live in the fur and feathers of animals and birds. Contrary to popular belief, most ticks do not carry disease. However, some of the buggers can transmit Lyme disease (caused by the organism *Borrelia burgdorferi*) and/or Rocky Mountain spotted fever.

Lyme disease is quite common in the eastern United States. Early symptoms of Lyme disease may include a red rash, possibly bull's-eye shaped, that appears an average of ten days after the bite (if it appears at all, and it doesn't in every case) and fades within a few weeks, even without treatment. Other signs include nonspecific flu-like symptoms such as profound fatigue, malaise, severe headache, fever, and severe muscle aches and pain.

Rocky Mountain spotted fever, originally diagnosed in the Northwest, is found in many parts of the United States. Symptoms of this condition include a sudden fever (which can last for two or three weeks), severe headache, tiredness, deep muscle pain, chills, nausea, and a characteristic rash. The rash might begin on the legs or arms, can include the soles of the feet or palms of the hands, and can spread rapidly to the trunk or the rest of the body.

The best preventive measure is to check yourself daily for ticks and pull them off immediately if you find them. A tick usually has to be attached for at least twenty-four hours in order to infect you with either of these diseases.

Mosquitoes

In the United States, mosquitoes were once known only as blood-sucking nuisances that left itchy welts behind. That changed a few years ago when a number of horses and birds were fatally infected with West Nile virus or WNV, which causes encephalitis (brain swelling) and sometimes death. Soon after, the first cases of human WNV in the United States were reported; according to the CDC, these cases grew from an initial outbreak of 62 in 1999 to 4,156, including 284 deaths, in 2002.

Although the statistics seem alarming, it's not easy to contract WNV. However, people with an impaired immune system such as the elderly, young children, and those with medically compromised immune function can be at risk. Early symptoms of WNV appear five to fifteen days after a bite. These symptoms may include severe headaches, fever, nausea and vomiting, disorientation, chills, muscle aches, pain, and/or stiffness, and require immediate medical attention.

If you're traveling in sub-Saharan Africa or tropical South America, be concerned with the mosquito species *Aedes aegypti*, as it transmits the viral illness called yellow fever. This disease can cause severe hepatitis and hemorrhagic fever, and, according to the CDC, can be deadly to those exposed. The most dangerous time of year for contracting yellow fever in West Africa is during the late rainy and early dry seasons (July–October); in Brazil, virus transmission is highest during the rainy season (January–March). Fortunately, there is a vaccination for yellow fever (see Chapter 1).

Another mosquito, the anopheles, transmits the parasite that causes malaria. Malaria affects the very small blood vessels of all the organs of the body, especially the brain, lungs, liver, and kidneys. It can occur in a mild form with recurring bouts of illness and fever. The severe form of malaria leads to coma, respiratory failure, kidney failure, and/or life-threatening blood sugar dysregulation, and has a high fatality rate. Considered one of the most common diseases throughout the world, malaria is most often found in the tropical climates of Mexico, Central and South America, Africa, Asia, and the Indian subcontinent (see Chapter 1).

There is presently no vaccine for malaria, but there are two major ways to prevent it: reduce your exposure to mosquitoes, and use chemoprophylaxis (that is, take an appropriate preventive drug before you are exposed to the disease-carrying mosquitoes). In deciding which drug you should use, your travel physician will consider several factors: your health, the region in which you are traveling, the type of parasite known to be endemic there, the length of your stay, and the climate, as well as the specific characteristics (and cost) of the drug.

Dengue fever is also transmitted by mosquito bite, usually during the day, especially in the two hours after sunrise and the two hours before sunset. It is primarily a disease of tropical climates, and most cases occur in crowded urban areas. Dengue causes a sudden onset of fever, severe headache, and internal bleeding. It can also cause shock, hemorrhage, and ultimately death.

There are several things you can do to help prevent mosquito stings, as follows:

- Use a DEET-containing insect repellent on your skin (see The Four D's on page 40).

- When you are outdoors, wear light-colored clothing with long pants and long sleeves.

- Use an insecticide such as permethrin on your clothes. (See the inset Buzz Off! on page 41.)

- Avoid perfumes, soaps, lotions, and hair products that contain floral fragrance.

- Use an insecticide spray to kill any indoor mosquitoes.

- Use insecticide-impregnated mosquito netting around your bed and around your child's stroller.

- Sleep in a well-closed room and above first-floor level, if possible.

In case any mosquitoes do breach your defenses and sting you, pack Benadryl for possible allergic reactions and pack a topical hydrocortisone cream or calamine lotion to soothe any itch.

Bees, Wasps, and Hornets, Oh My!

Although they love flowers and sweet summertime smells, stinging insects can be dangerous, especially for the millions of people allergic to bee, wasp, and hornet stings. These allergic reactions occur in two forms: a local reaction just causes swelling, pain, and itching at the site of the sting, whereas a systemic reaction causes hives, wheezing, swelling, difficulty breathing, and possibly death.

If you've had even a mild systemic reaction to an insect sting, get tested for the allergy before you travel and, if necessary, pack an epinephrine injection pen (EpiPen) to carry with you at all times. Don't wear bright clothing when you travel—and most importantly, don't panic and begin to swat!

Fire Ants

Fire ants, common throughout the southern part of the United States and countries south of the border, are very aggressive bugs that attack and sting anything that disturbs them. If you are stung, the burning and itching should subside within an hour but will likely be followed by blisters. Clean the stung area with soap and water to prevent infection, elevate it, and apply ice or a cold compress to reduce swelling and relieve pain. Allergic reactions are also possible. If you develop hives, swelling of the face, eyes, or throat, severe sweating, nausea, or difficulty breathing, seek medical attention immediately. Fire ant stings are not usually life threatening, but large numbers of fire ants attacking at once can cause death.

Kissing Bugs

Sounds cute, right? Don't be fooled. Reduviid bugs or "kissing bugs" are primarily found in South and Central America, living in cracks and holes of primitive or substandard housing. These insects become infected with the organism *Trypanosoma cruzi* after biting an animal or person who already has it. Chagas disease is spread to you when an infected reduviid bug deposits feces on your skin, usually while you're sleeping. You will become infected if you rub the feces into the bug-bite wound, an open cut, or your eyes or mouth (creating marks on your face that make it look like you've been kissed). Animals can become infected the same way, or by eating an infected bug.

According to the CDC, there are three phases of infection with Chagas disease (acute, indeterminate, and chronic), each with its own range of symptoms from fatigue and swollen glands to cardiac problems. Symptoms of the early acute stage can occur within a few days to weeks, but most people do not show symptoms until the later chronic stage—ten to twenty years after first being infected. Unfortunately, there is no vaccine. Medication to treat the disease does exist, but it must be given during the acute stage of infection for best effectiveness (and, as mentioned, that stage is typically asymptomatic).

Although Chagas disease may not affect the average traveler, it's still

important to know about the possible risk. The disease is locally transmitted in Argentina, Belize, Bolivia, Brazil, Chile, Colombia, Costa Rica,
Ecuador, El Salvador, French Guiana, Guatemala, Guyana, Honduras, Mexico, Nicaragua, Panama, Paraguay, Peru, Suriname, Uruguay, and Vene-
zuela. Blood supplies in some countries are not tested for *T. cruzi* and may
carry a risk of infection. The CDC stresses that travelers planning to stay in
hotels, resorts, or other well-constructed housing facilities are at less risk
for contracting the disease from reduviid bugs; as preventive measures
on your trip, use insecticides and do not sleep in thatch, mud, or adobe
houses.

The Four D's

"The best way to defend yourself from bugs is to remember the four D's:
dress, dawn, dusk, and DEET," according to Brawdy. "In highly infested
areas, you should wear light long pants and shirts and high socks too, and
tuck your clothes in, but since not many people really do this, you should
use insect repellent," he says. "Repellent is important because the experts
tell us to be careful at dawn and dusk because of bugs and don't go out
between 10:00 A.M. and 2:00 P.M. for sun, so if it were up to the experts, we
wouldn't be out much."

Insect repellent with a low concentration of diethyl-m-toluamide
(DEET) repels mosquitoes, ticks, and other biting bugs when applied to
skin. The higher the repellent's DEET concentration, the longer it will protect you, but you should only use a product with a maximum of 33 percent
DEET. You can also use an insecticide. Permethrin, for example, is a non-
toxic chemical that kills and repels mosquitoes, ticks, and other insects.
Permethrin-containing insecticides such as Permanone or deltamethrin
can be used directly on clothes or mosquito netting, but not on skin. Permethrin binds to fabric fibers and remains effective for up to six weeks,
even through washings, but should be reapplied after five washings.

COMMONSENSE TRAVEL TIPS

Here are some other suggestions to keep you healthy while traveling:

* Use condoms (latex condoms are best for disease protection unless you
  are allergic to latex). Unprotected sexual encounters can spread AIDS,
  hepatitis B, and other sexually transmitted diseases.

Buzz Off!

Check out Buzz Off insect-repellent travel apparel from Exofficio (www.exofficio.com) made with permethrin. The repellent is odorless and colorless, but the clothing is a bit pricey; it may be worth it, however, for people traveling to highly infested areas. Sample prices: hat $28, convertible pants $79, socks $18, long-sleeved shirt

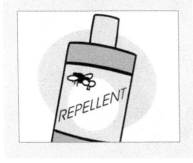

- If you are traveling internationally, do not walk barefoot, have any acupuncture or tattooing done, or pierce any body parts.

- If you are traveling internationally, and especially in tropical or subtropical countries, do not swim or wade or raft in freshwater, and do not walk barefoot on moist soil, or you risk contracting leptospirosis (mentioned earlier on page 28) or schistosomiasis (page 29). (See also Chapters 1 and 7 for information on other parasites and food-borne diseases.)

- Drink plenty of fluids to prevent heat-related illnesses such as heatstroke.

- "Slip, slop, slap!" The American Cancer Society wants you to remember slip, slop, and slap to protect your children from sunburn: slip on a shirt, slop on sunscreen, and slap on a hat to protect face, neck, and ears.

- Do not go out in the summer sun from 11:00 A.M. to 3:00 P.M. without adequate skin and eye protection. Wear a hat and a good pair of UV-protection sunglasses (with 99 to 100 percent ultraviolet A and B radiation protection), and frequently apply sunscreen with a sun-protection factor (SPF) of 15 or higher, especially to children, especially in summer and winter!

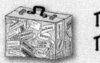

Traveler to Traveler

My travel credo: eat when you're hungry, drink when you're thirsty, and rest when you're tired. I try to make sure I don't get so swept up sightseeing or whatever that I ignore these simple objectives. It's so easy to get sick when you travel by getting sloppy about these basic habits.

—Sophia Dembling, freelance travel writer

About a week or so before you leave, add some yogurt to your diet. It will help to ward off intestinal illnesses.

—Pat Quaglieri

Pack thongs [flip-flops]! No matter how clean they are, I have a problem stepping into a hotel shower. Bring thongs or water shoes or something you can wear in the shower. Athlete's foot and other funguses can easily be caught in showers, and some funguses will never go away if they are contracted.

—Pat Quaglieri

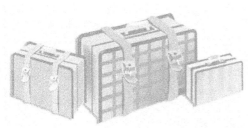

3. Traveler's Woes: DVT and Jet Lag

AHHH . . . . USING YOUR LONG FLIGHT TO GET OFF YOUR FEET and catch up on some sleep might seem like a good idea, but depending on your health and the length of your flight or ride, this kind of inactivity can disrupt your sleep/wake schedule—and could ultimately lead to a serious health problem.

CLOTTING AND EMBOLISM

Deep vein thrombosis or DVT is a serious medical condition that travelers should not ignore. DVT is inflammation and the development of a blood clot in a deep vein, usually in one of the lower extremities. It can also occur higher up the leg into the thigh and pelvic regions. (See Figure 3.1 on page 44.) The symptoms of DVT include pain, warmth, and swelling in the calf (or affected area), and pain while flexing the muscles in that area. It's important to know, however, that signs of DVT can appear up to several weeks after traveling, and that DVT can occur without symptoms as well.

In most cases, these clots can be treated with blood-thinning agents such as heparin and Coumadin, which prevent the formation of new clots and hopefully prevent the propagation or movement of clots already formed.

Whether or not there are any signs of DVT, an untreated clot can be transported through the blood-

Take Note!

If you develop calf pain and swelling at any time during your trip, seek immediate medical attention, especially if these symptoms are accompanied by shortness of breath and chest pain.

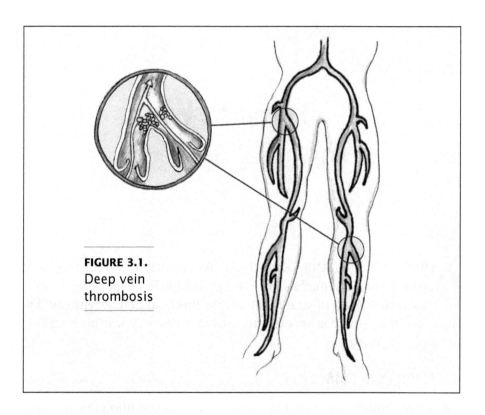

FIGURE 3.1.
Deep vein
thrombosis

stream to the lungs, where it becomes a pulmonary embolism or PE that can block off vital blood vessels. This will cause shortness of breath and chest pain that is made worse while breathing, and a PE can be fatal if not treated.

Startling Statistics

According to statistics found on the American Heart Association's website (www.preventdvt.org):

- Up to 2 million Americans are affected annually by DVT.

- Of those who develop a PE, up to 200,000 will die each year.

- More people die in the United States from a PE than from breast cancer, AIDS, and highway fatalities.

No study, however, shows exactly how many of these cases are caused by long travel.

Risk Factors

DVT was dubbed "economy class syndrome" when it was linked to restrictive legroom in airplanes. Although the stories of presumably healthy individuals who have died after a flight are frightening, there is no medical evidence that an airplane's cabin pressure and lack of fresh air contribute to DVT (low humidity, however, can cause dehydration, a known contributing factor in DVT). Remember that the most critical risk factor for getting a clot is immobility, so anything that causes the blood to sit and pool (such as riding in a car, train, bus, or plane for longer than three hours) could cause DVT.

Most travelers are *not* at risk of getting a blood clot, but certain people are more at risk. You are at "moderate" risk of getting a blood clot if you are:

- Over the age of sixty

- Obese

- A cardiovascular patient

- Pregnant (see Pregnancy, DVT, and PE on page 48)

- A smoker

- Using estrogen

- Diagnosed with a pronounced venous insufficiency

  Your risk increases to "high" if you have had:

- A previous diagnosis or treatment of DVT

- Surgery, especially of the lower extremities (for example, arthroscopic surgery or knee replacement)

- Serious or chronic illness

- Cancer

- A known predisposition to abnormal blood clotting

If you are at a moderate or high risk of developing DVT according to the factors mentioned above, or for any other reason, contact your doctor before traveling.

Airlines—British Airways was one of the first—are making a concerted effort to inform passengers of the potential risk of DVT on long flights and to provide tips for avoiding the condition. Some carriers such as Air New Zealand distribute leaflets about DVT; others such as Northwest Airlines and Qantas distribute health information and show aerobic videos on long flights, and recommend that passengers stretch and drink water every two hours.

Practical Precautions

To reduce your chances of developing blood clots while traveling, take the following simple steps:

- When making your seat selection, choose an exit row, a bulkhead seat, or an aisle seat for more legroom (see the Resources section at the back of the book for seat selection websites).

- Take walks both before and during the journey. If you're flying, walk around the airport as much as possible instead of lounging at the gate, and once on the plane, walk around as often as safety permits. If you're traveling by car, stop every few hours and take a walk; if traveling by bus or train, stroll around whenever possible and safe. If walking opportunities are limited by turbulence, crowding, or other constraints, move your legs in your seat every fifteen minutes.

- Stretch during the journey. To increase blood flow to your calves, stand on your toes or do toe-lifts in your seat. Loosen your ankles by pointing and flexing your toes and rotating your feet in circles. (See also the inset Yoga! on page 47.)

- Don't cross your legs. It shortens the leg muscles, reduces circulation, and creates an uneven weight distribution on the hips and pelvis, which can cause pain in the lower back.

- Wear loose-fitting clothes. Avoid girdles and avoid socks or stockings with tight elastic bands below the knee.

- Wear some form of elasticized support on your calves to prevent blood from settling in the veins in your legs. (See the inset Buying Compression Stockings on page 48.)

- Drink lots of water during and after the trip. Avoid caffeine and alcohol. Don't smoke.

- Check with your doctor about taking an aspirin or even an anticoagulant medication as a precautionary blood-thinner a few days before and after your long-distance flight. *Note:* The benefit of aspirin against DVT is not proven, and in some people aspirin can affect the stomach by causing irritation (gastritis) and possibly bleeding.

If the flight or ride is less than six hours long and you do not have any of the risk factors mentioned previously, then you needn't take specific preventive measures beyond regularly moving your feet and legs and drinking plenty of fluids. But if the flight or ride is more than six hours (especially if it's more than twelve) and/or you are at moderate or high risk for DVT, further precautions are advised. Discuss the situation with your physician ahead of time, including the possible prophylactic use of an anticoagulant. While *en route*, make sure to wear compression stockings, frequently move your feet and legs, walk around whenever possible, and drink an abundance of liquids (avoiding alcohol and caffeine).

Yoga!

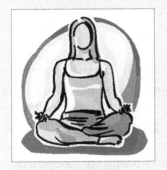

"Here's a great yoga exercise that you can do right in your chair, to help get circulation going and muscles moving. Spinal twists are invigorating and balancing, and easy to do almost anywhere—they're great when you're starting to feel stiff in the middle of a long plane ride. Sit straight near the front edge of your chair with your thighs parallel and feet flat on the floor. Place your left hand on your left thigh. As you breathe out, move just the upper part of your body to the right and place your right hand on the back of your chair. Relax, and breathe into the twist for several breaths. Repeat on the opposite side." (From an interview with Lynn Ginsburg and Mary Taylor, authors of *What Are You Hungry For? Women, Food and Spirituality*, New York, NY: St. Martin's Griffin Press, 2003; www.whatareyouhungryfor.net.)

Buying Compression Stockings

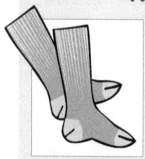 Compression stockings, also called support socks, are designed to help prevent blood from pooling in the feet and legs. They are put on first thing in the morning before getting out of bed (before swelling starts), and are removed only for bathing and for sleeping at night. Compression stockings typically cover the area from the arch of the foot to just below or just above the knee. They are tightest at the foot, and the tightness gradually lessens from the ankle toward the top of the stocking.

With a doctor's prescription, you can buy compression stockings from a medical supply store. They may cost from $60 to $100 a pair (pantyhose styles are more expensive). Check your insurance plan, as some cover compression stockings in the category of "durable medical equipment." You can also buy them without a prescription, but the level of compression may not be as high as with prescription stockings. For more information, visit the following websites: www.supportsockshop.com, www.magellans.com, and www.footsmart.com.

Pregnancy, DVT, and PE

According to the website www.preventdvt.org, a woman's risk of developing DVT is six times greater during pregnancy, and PE is the leading cause of maternal death associated with childbirth, so moms-to-be need to be particularly careful about preventing DVT. Pregnancy-related changes in blood-clotting factors, venous dilation, and/or partial venous obstruction put pregnant travelers at risk for superficial and deep thrombophlebitis (inflammation of a vein), especially on flights longer than six hours.

Because sitting for prolonged periods can significantly increase DVT risk, pregnant women should limit their seated travel to a maximum of six hours per day. If you are going to be a pregnant passenger, talk with your obstetrician about using compression stockings. You should make a point of taking frequent walks around the cabin and doing some basic stretching exercises (being careful during turbulence, of course). It's also very important to drink large amounts of nonalcoholic/non-caffeinated beverages to compensate for water loss from the extremely low humidity on pressurized flights.

JET LAG

Writer Pat Curry travels on business and for fun, but it leaves her exhausted. "I am just wiped out," says Curry. "I'm waking up at 3:00 or 4:00 in the morning and falling asleep during dinner. When I went to Durban, South Africa, the flight over was horrible (tiny seats for fourteen hours) and I really can't sleep on an airplane, so I was very tired. We got in early afternoon and I just had to take a nap."

Has flying made you tired, bleary eyed, out of sorts, and needing a few days to recover from your trip? If so, you've had jet lag. In a nutshell, jet lag occurs when your body clock (the regulator of your circadian rhythms) is thrown out of whack by quickly changing time zones. It causes such symptoms as decreased awareness, general sleepiness and/or fatigue, impaired mental ability and memory, headaches, stomachaches, and other discomforts such as cramps, diarrhea, and constipation, reduced physical activity and energy, and irritability.

The Root of the Problem

When you travel to a different time zone by bus, car, boat, or train, your body has a chance to slowly adjust by the time you reach your destination. When you fly, however, you pass through time zones so quickly that your body clock cannot adapt swiftly enough from its original schedule to a new one. For example, let's say you fly from San Diego to New York City and have an 8:00 A.M. appointment the next morning. Why do you end up struggling to keep your eyes open through the meeting? Because your internal clock is still on California time, which is three hours earlier than New York time—so you feel like the meeting is actually taking place at 5:00 A.M.! And when you hit the sack in New York at 11:00 P.M. for some much-needed shut-eye, you can't sleep, because in California it is only 8:00 P.M.

If you fly across only one or two time zones, you may be able to make the adjustment with minimal side effects. If you cross three or more time zones, however, you may be more vulnerable to symptoms of jet lag. Generally, the symptoms are worst when you travel from west to east, and less bothersome when you travel from east to west (this is because our biological clock has an innate tendency to run on a daily cycle that is actually

A Good Ol' Dose of Sunshine

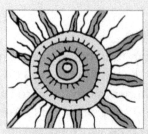 "The importance of light to human health is one of those facts that everyone once knew and then somehow forgot. Florence Nightingale, the foremother of modern nursing, asserted that patients' faces should be turned toward the light. She campaigned for sunrooms and open windows in hospitals. Researchers at the University of Alberta in Edmonton, Canada recently affirmed her bright idea. They found that getting a sunny room rather than a dull one boosts odds of survival in persons admitted to the hospital after suffering heart attacks. It also helps those with depression recover sooner." (From *The Body Clock Guide to Better Health*, page 34.)

longer than twenty-four hours, which makes it easier to reset when going "backward" in time rather than "forward"). If you travel strictly north to south or south to north, jet lag isn't an issue, because you don't cross any time zones.

Fortunately, according to Lynne Lamberg, coauthor of *The Body Clock Guide to Better Health* (with Michael Smolensky, Ph.D., New York, NY: Henry Holt & Company, 2000), "With advance planning and attention to how you organize your day in a new time zone, you can avoid many of the unpleasant consequences of jet lag."

Chronobiology to the Rescue

Chronobiology, the study of the body's internal clock and rhythms, is rapidly gaining recognition in the medical community. But according to Lamberg, "Most doctors, even those who claimed to know something about chronobiology, did not know that some common illnesses predictably flare in the morning, afternoon, evening, or night." Research shows, for example, that heart attacks and strokes most commonly occur early in the morning. The body clock's influence is also evident in the timing of conception. Ovulation kits monitor the cyclic changes in hormones and temperature that determine a woman's most fertile time of the month.

"Sunlight keeps most of us synchronized with the local twenty-four-hour day," explains Lamberg. "Studies have shown that the control of body rhythms comes from within but responds to time cues in the environment, most notably, light." Within a brain structure called the hypothalamus, which regulates breathing, heart rate, temperature, blood pressure, hormone production, and various other bodily functions, is the body clock's main control mechanism: the suprachiasmatic nucleus or SCN. Through signals received from the eyes' optic nerves, the SCN monitors environmental light, and in turn regulates certain body responses in accordance with the light level.

Travelers can benefit from chronobiology by using sunlight (or certain forms of bright artificial light) to beat jet lag. The amount of light you should get depends largely on the length of your stay. For example, if you are staying more than a few days, follow the time schedule of your new destination immediately, and be sure to get as much sun as you can. On the other hand, if you are not staying in your new time zone for more than a day or so, chronobiology experts suggest avoiding sunlight as much as possible so that your rhythms *don't* shift; instead, eat and sleep according to the schedule that you'll be returning to shortly. Why? Because the struggle to reset your rhythms during a short trip can become a vicious cycle: by the time you adjust to the new time frame at your destination, it's probably time to fly back to where you came from, and then your body clock must adjust once again to the old time frame. Some travelers take days to recover from all of this internal effort once they're home.

Counteracting jet lag with exposure to bright light isn't just a question of *how much* you get, but also of *when* you get it. Visit www.bodyclock.com and use the website's Jetlag calculator before your trip. You'll need to answer two questions: How many time zones does your journey cover? What time do you regularly go to sleep? The site will then create instructions for you on when to seek and avoid bright light to help reduce jet lag symptoms.

The Circadian Lighting Association (CLA) is an international group of manufacturers who supply artificial light sources specially designed for circadian applications including combating severe jet lag, improving winter mood, and treating the form of depression known as seasonal affective disorder or SAD. The website www.claorg.org describes four basic portable, lightweight alternatives: a light box, a visor (a head-mounted light source that looks something like a tennis visor, good for traveling), a bright desk lamp (functions much like a light box), and a dawn simulator (mimics natural sunrise, gradually brightening a room over a set time period). Each

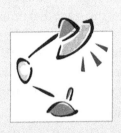

Artificial Light Sources

The CLA recommends the manufacturers listed below. Before purchasing any artificial light source, make certain that you visit the company's website to know what you're looking for and what questions to ask.

Apollo Light Systems	Enviro-Med, Inc.	Outside In
Orem, UT, USA	Vancouver, WA, USA	Cambridge, UK, Europe
800-545-9667	800-222-DAWN	+ 44 (0)1954 780 500
www.apollolight.com	www.bio-light.com	www.outsidein.co.uk
Bio-Brite, Inc.	Northern Light	SunBox Co.
Bethesda, MD, USA	Montreal, Canada	Gaithersburg, MD, USA
800-621-LITE	800-263-0066	800-548-3968
www.biobrite.com	www.northernlight-tech.com	www.sunboxco.com

device has pros and cons that you should evaluate in the context of your own needs and situation. For purchasing information, see the above inset on Artificial Light Sources.

More Strategies for Coping with Jet Lag

Is every traveler who flies doomed to suffer from jet lag? Not necessarily. Following are some preventive tips from the National Sleep Foundation (www.sleepfoundation.org):

- Anticipate the upcoming time change for at least several days prior to your journey by getting up and going to bed earlier for an eastward trip, later for a westward trip.

- Select a flight that allows early evening arrival.

- Upon boarding the plane, set your watch to your destination's time zone.

- While *en route,* avoid alcohol and caffeine for at least three to four hours before bedtime (both act as stimulants and interfere with sleep).

- Upon arrival at your destination, avoid heavy meals. A snack—not chocolate, it's caffeinated—is okay.

- Avoid any heavy exercise close to bedtime. Light exercise earlier in the day, however, is fine.

- Once at your destination, stay up until 10:00 P.M. local time.

- Bring earplugs and an eye mask or blindfold to dampen noise and block out light while sleeping.

- If you must sleep during the day, take a short nap in the early afternoon, but no longer than two hours, and set an alarm so as not to oversleep.

Are you traveling across many time zones, perhaps even ten or more? It might be beneficial, if possible, to break your trip into stages—an especially important consideration if you have frequently had severe jet lag. For example, you may want to stay over for a few days in a city or town that's about halfway along your route. This will give your body some time to adjust before you reach your final destination, and any symptoms of jet lag that you may experience should not be as strong.

Meditation to "Reset" Yourself

If you're one of the unlucky people hit hard by jet lag, you can fight it off by using several other methods. Jerry V. Teplitz, Ph.D., a professional speaker for more than thirty years, has created a CD called *Travel Stress* (www.teplitz.com). "In chatting with other speakers, I noticed they were fried energetically, but I wasn't," says Teplitz. "I started thinking about that more and realized that my stress-management techniques were keeping *me* from getting stressed out."

When Teplitz flies, he makes sure to perform two meditations while on the plane (more on long flights). "When you meditate, you go into a state of rest or relaxation, and you're setting your biorhythms very quickly in that process. When I had flown from Virginia to Australia, I meditated and slept, then did a full afternoon seminar for four hours. They were amazed, and had no idea that I had just flown in." How does Teplitz meditate? "Just make your mind go blank, and don't get upset about thoughts when you have them. Just have them and move on."

Melatonin and Other Supplements

Of the many products on the market that purport to fight jet lag, melatonin is one of the most popular and controversial. Melatonin, a hormone

Homeopathic Help

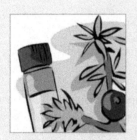

Stevanne Auerbach, Ph.D., also known as "Dr. Toy," travels more than 100,000 miles in a year in search of toys and educational products for kids, and she is all too familiar with jet lag. "I take homeopathic products, such as No Jet-Lag made in New Zealand, that help with the symptoms, but coming back, it always takes time for my body to adjust again," says Auerbach.

We do not have any medical information on No Jet-Lag, but we've heard travelers swear by its effectiveness, and the product's website www.nojetlag.com features many positive anecdotal testimonies. If you choose to try it, please let your travel physician know, and notify him/her of any other medications and/or supplements you are taking.

normally produced in the brain by the pineal gland, plays a role in regulating our daily sleep/wake cycle. Some studies have shown that small doses of melatonin can improve sleep. Studies have also shown, however, that taking too much melatonin or taking it at the wrong time can actually disrupt the sleep/wake cycle or cause other side effects such as confusion, drowsiness, and headache.

Advocates of taking melatonin claim that it influences the body clock and eases symptoms of jet lag. Dr. Andrew Weil, renowned author of eight books including the national bestsellers *Spontaneous Healing, Eight Weeks to Optimum Health,* and *Eating Well for Optimum Health,* takes melatonin when he travels. He writes, "In general, I have found that, after arriving at my destination, taking 1 milligram of melatonin sublingually [under the tongue] at bedtime for only one or two nights significantly reduces jet lag, regardless of the direction of travel" (www.drweil.com).

Melatonin is available over the counter and marketed as a dietary supplement. Unlike drugs, supplements are not regulated by the FDA, so a manufacturer doesn't need to prove them safe or effective. Hormones sold as dietary supplements may therefore not be as thoroughly studied as drugs are, so their potential consequences and their influence on health (particularly when taken over a long period of time) may be unknown; in addition, they may interfere with other medications. For these reasons, the

National Institute on Aging (www.nia.nih.gov) warns consumers against taking melatonin or any supplement without consulting a physician.

The Argonne Anti-Jet-Lag Diet

Although it is popularly believed that the *types* of foods we eat can affect jet lag symptoms for better or for worse, scientific research has not yet definitively refuted or supported this idea. You might, however, be able to "eat your way through jet lag" by using the Argonne Anti-Jet-Lag Diet, which was developed by Dr. Charles F. Ehret in the Division of Biological and Medical Research at Argonne National Laboratory (one of the U.S. Department of Energy's major centers of research) as an application of his fundamental studies on the daily biological rhythms of animals.

This diet is actually "a coordinated plan that combines a number of time-giving cues—including alternate days of moderate feasting and fasting—to help speed your adjustment to a new schedule. Still, we call it a 'diet' because meals are central. What you eat sends your body signals about waking up and going to sleep. And because meals tend to occur at reasonably consistent times during the day, their regularity helps to reinforce the regularity of other time-setting activities. The Anti-Jet-Lag Diet can help prevent jet lag with a planned rescheduling of time-giving cues. It starts a few days ahead of your departure date to prepare your time zone adjustment by carefully planning the amounts and types of food eaten at meal times. On the day you arrive at your destination, your body's clock is reset by assuming the same meal and activity schedule as people in the new time zone." (Visit www.antijetlagdiet.com/index.asp for more information.)

Anti-Jet Lag Accommodations

Recognition of jet lag's impact on travelers is spreading, and the travel industry (astutely) wants to help combat jet lag and its symptoms. Hilton Hotels (www.hilton.com), for example, has introduced rooms featuring sleep products such as a sunrise clock (it simulates dawn) and a light box to help realign the body's circadian rhythms to the local time zone. For travelers who need shut-eye assistance, The Marriott's Courtyard Hotel at the Warsaw International Airport Hotel (www.marriott.com) provides tips for restful slumber and also a complimentary jet lag recovery menu of amenities including an eye mask to block out light, soothing lavender aromatherapy oil to restore and rebalance mind and body, and—last but not least—a warm glass of milk delivered bedside as a nightcap.

The ten Stamford Hotels and Resorts located throughout Australia in Sydney, Adelaide, Auckland, Brisbane, and Melbourne offer a jet lag recovery package that features early check-in and late check-out to accommodate flight times, particularly international arrivals and departures as well as the infamous "Perth red-eye" frequented by many business travelers. Along with free pressing of clothing (three items per person), guests also receive a Jet Lag Recovery Kit containing unisex Caire facial mist, hydration gel, moisture silk, and lip silk, specially formulated by Aire Natural Science Labs to reduce the effects of jet lag and dehydration caused by flying and air conditioning. (The package is subject to advance booking and availability, and conditions apply; call 800-223-5652, or 300-301-391 when in Australia, or visit the website www.stamford.com.au.)

These three programs are just a sample of a growing trend. Ask whether your hotel offers any special services or amenities to help travelers with jet lag.

 Traveler to Traveler

I travel trans-Pacific flights frequently. I don't use anything [to combat jet lag], but I do time my activities. I pick flights that arrive in the afternoon or early evening whenever possible. A day or so before leaving, I start eating less of everything and drinking more water. The night before flying, I stay up later than usual and get up earlier so I know I'll want to take a nap at some point. Upon arrival, I get active with a long walk or a swim, do lots of stretches, and stay up past my bedtime. Before going to sleep, I make a cup of laxative tea to combat fourteen-plus hours of pressurized air and to force regularity on local time. I know it sounds crazy, but it has worked for me for years.

—Beth Hughes

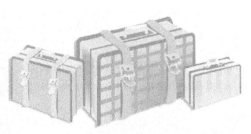

4. Lines, Luggage, and Screaming Children: Stress-Free Travel Is Possible!

T RAVELING IS MEANT TO BE FUN, ENJOYABLE, AND ADVENTURESOME. At times, a journey can even be a relief from the daily grinds of housework, kids, work, bills, and problems. Unfortunately, security checkpoints, delayed flights, lost luggage, traffic jams, and hearing "Are we there yet?" at regular intervals can knot the stomachs of even the most relaxed travelers.

Preventing bumps along the way requires some planning before you even board the plane, step on the train, or get in the car—from the moment you know that you want or need to go somewhere. In addition to taking the necessary steps to minimize the stress and maximize the pleasure, stress-free traveling also means being flexible and having a positive attitude in handling any obstacles, foreseen or not. As Winston Churchill once said, "Attitude is a little thing that makes a big difference."

WHAT IS BUGGING YOU?

First, you need to figure out what stresses you out. Is it the planning: surfing the Web for the best deals, working with travel agents, packing, or tracking vital pre-trip details? Perhaps traveling with the kids tenses you up: bickering between siblings, incessant (and often expensive) requests for souvenirs, or whining, tired children? Maybe you love to travel but have a hard time sleeping in an unfamiliar bed?

Next, make a list of your travel-related annoyances—as many as you can identify—so you can pinpoint what needs your attention. (*Note:* This is even more important if you are traveling with any preexisting medical conditions that are associated with stress-related flare-ups: for example, acid reflux disease, arthritis, Crohn's disease, diabetes, irritable bowel syndrome, or a major personality disorder, among others. See also Chapters 1 and 3.) Repeat this list-making process before each trip, in case something new arises.

Hopefully, this chapter will cover all of your travel stressors, and by the time you are done reading it, you will have learned how to eliminate them. If there is something on your list that we haven't addressed, ponder what additional strategies you can implement to make that part of your trip more enjoyable. Keep this book or a copy of Chapter 10's handy checklists in your carry-on bag, so you can use them as you go and update them regularly for future stress-free travel.

Planning + Spontaneity = Stress-Free Travel

You might want to create a daily itinerary for your trip, especially if you are making all the plans yourself, but be sure not to overschedule the days—and have backup options in case something falls through. Expecting the unexpected and knowing how to enjoy the spontaneous are key to keeping your stress level at bay.

Stress Factor #1:
Booking It, Danno!

Should you use a travel agent to book your trip, or make the arrangements yourself? The method you choose depends on your personality, your level of patience, and the time available.

Travel agents are knowledgeable industry professionals who can provide one-stop, stress-free vacation planning, handling everything from booking flights and cruises to planning activities and tours. If you can't spare the time (or tolerate the occasional tedium) to research your trip on the Web, compare prices, and find out whether your membership in the American Automobile Association (AAA; www.aaa.com) entitles you to any discounts, a travel agent can design a travel package based on your specifications and do the legwork for you. Make sure your agent compares the prices of several airlines and hotels. Some agents focus only on specific airlines and hotels, which won't always get you the lowest fares or rates.

Doing It Yourself: Lisa's Experience

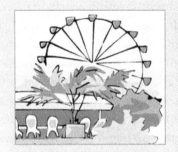

Although an agent can save you time and money, you may save even more money yourself if you're a smart shopper. For example, for a trip with my parents and three children, I compared prices at popular travel websites and read articles on vacationing at Disney. In *Budget Travel* magazine, I read about a hotel outside Disney that offered a significantly reduced rate for grandparents traveling with grandchildren. I did more research to organize the rest of the trip, and can confidently say that I saved hundreds of dollars compared to the travel agent's quote—some details were different, but staying under budget certainly relieved some of *my* stress! It took time, but it was a task that I enjoyed. If I were traveling to an unfamiliar destination, however, I would prefer to leave this work to an agent. I know my own patience level, and I know when to defer to others for their expertise.

For help finding a travel agent near you, visit the American Society of Travel Agents website at www.astanet.com (you can search by zip code). Word of mouth, of course, is the best way to find an agent who did a terrific job for someone else, so ask your friends and family for recommendations. Ask the travel agent how long he/she's been in the business, and check his/her certification. Membership in professional travel agency associations is a plus. An agent with at least five years' experience can also complete a two-year graduate program offered by the Institute of Certified Travel Agents (www.icta.com) to earn the qualification of Certified Travel Counselor or CTC.

Stress Factor #2: The "Ack" in Packing

Life is funny to humor writer Michele Wojciechowski (www.wojos world.com), but packing for a trip is not. "Packing stressed me out the most," says Michele. "I was always panicked that I would forget something—things that I may not usually think of, like taking one sweatshirt in the summer in case the weather gets cold, or bringing medicine for mosquito bites. Sure, sometimes you can buy the stuff you need wherever you're staying, but sometimes you can't."

So Michele made packing a serious business, creating a personalized packing list on her computer. "Before each trip, I print it out—the list includes everything from clothing to toiletries," she says. "My husband and I cross it off as we pack it. This eliminates forgetting major items and has really decreased our pre-trip stress. I update the list after each trip." If you haven't already prepared a list of your own, don't worry. We've created a comprehensive travel checklist for you (see Chapter 10), which includes packing lists for your checked luggage and carry-on bag—along with other lists to help you take care of everything else you have to do before your trip. A guiding principle: pack as lightly as possible. Remember, you will be carrying it, so think about what is most important.

Have You Considered Luggage-Free Travel?

Toting suitcases, golf clubs, a laptop, food, and a child through the airport can be stressful, cumbersome, and a pain in the back. You can forgo haul-ing extra gear yourself, or even ship all of your luggage, through companies such as Luggage Concierge (www.luggageconcierge.com), Golf Bag Shipping (www.golfbagshipping.com), or Luggage Free (www.luggagefree.com). In short, the company picks up your bags from your home, delivers them to your destination, and, if you order a return package, picks the bags up again from that destination and returns them to your home. Ta-da! Trav-elers who use these services are provided with special heavy-duty plastic shipping bags in which to seal their luggage and identify it with specially supplied labels. Once the luggage arrives safely, the clients are notified by their choice of email, fax, or phone.

At press time, one-way shipping of a golf bag and a small suitcase from New York to California costs $188.00 at Golf Bag Shipping; round-trip delivery through Luggage Concierge is nearly $400; and the minimum order for Luggage Free is $95 for luggage and $135 for sports equipment, inclusive of a $20 pick-up fee within twenty miles of the airport. Granted, this kind of service is a tad pricey, but it can save you a whole lot of stress and time at security checks and luggage pick-up areas. (Compare these prices to the cost of packaging and shipping the items via your local post office—make sure a return site is available.)

You may be able to maximize your frequent-traveler benefits to mini-mize your schlepping. Fairmont Hotels and Resorts, for example, has partnered with Sports Express to bring guests of the Fairmont President's Club Program nationwide a complete door-to-door solution for the delivery of luggage and sports equipment via shipping carrier (www.fairmont.com/fpc/SportsExpress). Or, if you often stay at the same hotel, ask the staff if you can leave your luggage behind. The Four Seasons in Washington, D.C. (www.fourseasons.com/washington) offers TravelLight exclusively to its most frequent guests. You leave your garment bag with the hotel when you depart, laundry or dry-cleaning services are provided upon request for any clothing, and your personal items are secured. The next time you arrive, your clothes are hanging in the closet, your shoes are freshly polished, and your personal items are waiting in your room. (If anything is lost, the hotel will assist in replacing it.) This program is *great* for frequent business travelers!

Stress Factor #3: "We're Sorry, But We Don't Have Your Reservation—OR Your Luggage."

This is probably one of the most frustrating things a traveler can hear. It is *very* important to carry copies of *any and all* reservations you made through a travel agent, tour operator, or the Internet. Print out any details including confirmation numbers and payment information.

As for your luggage—if you aren't traveling luggage free, that is!—first make sure to tag it properly, and put your name and your destination address inside (*not* your home address). Second, pack as though you *are* going to lose your luggage. Does this sound crazy? Maybe, but if you're heading to Australia and your bags are heading to China, at least you'll have your necessities and valuables on you. Don't pack cash, important documents, medication, or anything valuable in your checked luggage: pack these things in your carry-on bag, along with a change of clothes. (See also Traveler to Traveler tips on page 73.)

Stress Factor #4: Security Lines

In this era of heightened security, you need to expect delays. The key to saving time in security screening is spending a little extra prep time before you get to the airport. The Transportation Security Administration (TSA; www.tsa.gov) provides the following suggestions to reduce your wait time:

Before the Airport

- Do *not* pack or bring prohibited items to the airport. Check the list of

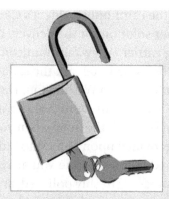

Lock It Up

The list below identifies luggage locks that are "accepted and recognized" by the TSA, which means that TSA screeners have the tools to open and relock them without damaging them or cutting the lock if a physical inspection is required. Some of the locks listed are specific brands, whereas others are manufacturers that produce a wide variety of locks, only some of which are compatible with TSA screeners' tools. If you plan on using a luggage lock for air travel, check the packaging to ensure that it has language similar to "accepted and recognized by TSA" (most locks on the market, in fact, are not TSA recognized). Before you travel, check the TSA's website for an updated list of accepted and recognized brands.

- American Tourister Accessories
- Atlantic Luggage
- Austin House Travel Essentials
- Brookstone Easy Check
- Eagle Creek Travel Safe
- EasyGo
- eBags
- Franzus Travel Smart
- Lewis N. Clark
- Master Lock
- Prestolock SearchAlert
- Royal Traveler by Samsonite Accessories
- Samsonite Accessories
- Samsonite Luggage
- Sharper Image
- Target Embark
- Voltage Valet

If it is necessary to open a bag, TSA screeners will always strive to do so without breaking the lock, and they do have the ability to open luggage and/or locks not listed above. Time pressures, however, may occasionally require cutting the locks rather than sorting through the many manufacturers' multiple master keys. It is very important to the TSA that your baggage makes it onto your plane, and screeners will do everything possible to balance security needs with customer service considerations.

these items online at www.tsa.gov/public/interapp/editorial/editorial_1012.xml.

- Place valuables such as jewelry, laptop computers, and cash in your carry-on bag only.

- Avoid wearing shoes, clothing, jewelry, and other accessories that contain metal, as these may set off the alarm on the metal detector.

- Put all undeveloped film and cameras containing film in your carry-on bag, as the screening equipment used on checked baggage will damage undeveloped film.

- Declare firearms and ammunition to your airline and pack them in your checked baggage.

- If you wish to lock your baggage, use a TSA-recognized lock (see inset on page 62).

At the Airport

- Keep available the airline boarding pass and government-issued photo ID (such as a driver's license) for each adult traveler until you exit the security checkpoint.

- Place the following items in your carry-on bag prior to entering the screening checkpoint: cell phones, keys, loose change, money clips, personal digital assistant (PDA), lighters, large amounts of jewelry, metal hair decorations, large belt buckles.

- Take your laptop out of its case.

- Take off any outer jackets (you do not have to remove your sport jacket).

Be sure to check the TSA's website (www.tsa.gov) before you leave for the most up-to-date information.

Stress Factor #5: White Knuckles and High Anxiety

Nothing makes stress levels soar higher than the fear of flying. According to psychotherapist and author Tina Tessina, Ph.D. (www.tinatessina.com), fear of flying is usually the result of negative "self-talk" that exaggerates the dangers of flight. "Sometimes it is caused by a bad experience such as having a friend or family member who was in an airplane accident, or experiencing a very turbulent flight," says Dr. Tessina. "Even the 9/11 TV coverage can induce flying anxiety."

To cope with the anxiety, she suggests desensitization. "First, learn a relaxation technique, such as deep breathing, self-hypnosis, or meditation," she says. "When you have learned to relax yourself and turn off the mental 'chatter,' try picturing an airplane trip, and stop the mental picture at each step of the way (packing luggage, driving to airport, entering airport, checking bags, entering airplane, taking off, in flight, landing). Calm yourself down using your relaxation technique. Do this repeatedly until you can get all the way through an imaginary flight without anxiety. Then, ask a calm friend to go with you to the airport (at a time when you're not flying) and do the relaxation steps again, in the actual airport. Once you can stay calm doing this, then try a short flight, preferably with the same calm friend."

Dr. Tessina offers several other tips to help decrease flying anxiety, as follows:

- Take a tape player or CD player and headphones to play soothing music or a self-hypnosis tape during the flight.

- Bring a book-on-tape or a handheld solitaire game to keep yourself busy.

- Stay away from newscasts and television programs about flight accidents. If necessary, get your news from the written word (which doesn't have the hyper-anxious feel of televised news) so you can manage what you take in.

- Being well rested and properly fed will enhance your ability to calm yourself.

Sheila Delson, president of FREEDomain Concepts in Poughkeepsie, New York, considers herself a "high-anxiety flyer" but has to fly several times a year on business as a professional organizer. Through the years, Delson has experimented with several coping strategies to make her flights less stressful. "First, twenty minutes before the flight, I take an over-the-counter herbal product to relax me," she says. "Next, I remind myself that I am going on this plane voluntarily. I am not a victim, and I must release myself to the experience I committed to. I bring along a good book and chewing gum as tension releasers. Between the herbal product, the book, the self-talk, and gum, I am now able to settle down, and sometimes I even nap! I still do not like to fly, but it gets me from here to there, and it sure is better than it used to be."

To assess your degree of fear of flying, visit the website of the Institute of Psychology for Air Travel at www.fearlessflying.net, where you can click on the test, answer the questions, and add up your score. If your score is high, consider participating in a fear-of-flying treatment program. The site lists programs available in the United States and worldwide.

If you don't have a fear of flying, but your anxiety level climbs a few points when the jet engines rev up, there are a number of things you can do to help stay relaxed. See what works best for you among the following:

- Eat a well-balanced meal, pack healthful snacks for the flight, and stay hydrated.

- Get a good sleep the night before you travel.

- Anxiety is often the result of stress and a feeling of being overwhelmed. Last-minute packing and rushing to the airport can contribute to your anxiety, so leave time to pack and travel to the airport without hitting rush-hour traffic.

- Tell your flight crew how you are feeling. This is especially helpful if you are uneasy because you're flying for the first time. Once you've gotten

Looks Odd, But It Works: Reflexotherapy

Waiting in long lines, sitting for extended periods, and sleeping in unfamiliar and/or uncomfortable beds can lead to travel's common side effects of muscle tension and discomfort. Try using the Reflexotherapy Applicator offered by Dynamic Pain Relief (www.dynamicpainrelief.com), founded by Irene Tamaras to provide alternative self-help treatments and products after she suffered a severe back injury twelve years ago that led to chronic back pain. The Reflexotherapy Applicator ($79.95) rolls up to fit in a suitcase. If you're not familiar with acupuncture or reflexology, its prickly points may intimidate you, but Tamaras claims it can help relieve insomnia, migraines and other headaches, and neck pain.

(Author's note: I love massages but can't always have one while traveling, so I tried this unique device on my upper back, and I did feel less tense afterward. —Lisa) your nervousness off your chest, the flight attendants can then check on you periodically to offer additional water and snacks and reassure you that you're doing fine.

- Bring a favorite item from home to keep yourself busy or relaxed: a CD, book, magazine, or even work.

- Take deep breaths and count to ten each time you feel some anxiety coming on, and move around the cabin when the conditions permit.

Ask your airline what they have to help you relax in flight. Virgin Atlantic (www.virgin-atlantic.com), for example, offers in-flight massages and beauty treatments, and has even introduced in-flight hypnotherapists who offer various services such as making you believe the flight lasts only a few minutes or that you are sitting next to your favorite celebrity!

Stress Factor #6: Delays and Layovers

Stuck on a four-hour layover, or unexpectedly delayed at the airport? Skip the watering hole! Today's airports offer a surprising array of diversions from spa treatments to art exhibits, so you can use this extra time to relax and rejuvenate. The key is to check the airport's website before your trip. You'll be surprised to see how a little bit of research can turn "downtime" into a fun experience for everybody.

To help take out those traveling kinks, try the instant massage tables and assorted spa treatments at the Philadelphia Airport and Detroit Metropolitan Airport. Aquamassage, an increasingly popular alternative to traditional massage, combines hydro-therapy and dry-heat therapy. You lie in the machine while dozens of water-jets, enclosed in a waterproof mantle, soothe or invigorate you for five to twenty minutes (and you don't get wet!). The wellness spa Oraoxygen is

Wireless Airport Info

From your PDA or cell phone, you can go to the website www.faa.gov/wireless for up-to-the-minute information on any delays, ground stops, or weather problems at your air-port(s) of interest—you can even check the status of your specific flight.

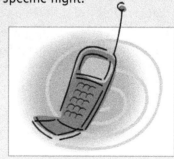

equipped with an oxygen bar, showers, and body treatments. At New York's JFK International Airport, the Oasis Day Spa for JetBlue Airways' passengers features two treatment rooms for massages, facials, and other salon services.

Enjoy a stroll through "terminal culture"! Artists and gallery curators now display an infinite variety of paintings, sculptures, fabric art, and photographs in permanent and rotating exhibits at terminals worldwide. Amsterdam's Schiphol Airport, for example, opened a branch of the world-renowned Rijksmuseum with paintings by old masters such as Rembrandt, Jan Steen, and Peter de Hooch. The San Francisco International Airport, among others, commissions the works of local artists to showcase regional flavor to visitors. And Milwaukee's General Mitchell International Airport is home to the Mitchell Gallery of Flight, an aviation museum.

Did you know that California's Palm Springs International Airport has an indoor putting green? Or that you can enjoy some self-reflection time at the San Francisco Airport's Berman Reflection Room (located at the International Terminal Main Hall)? If you have little ones, don't worry, the airport is not just an adult's playground. Many airports now offer arcade games and indoor playrooms to help tots expend their extra energy.

Stress Factor #7: Sleepless in Seattle . . . or Elsewhere

There's no place like home, and snoozing isn't always easy when you're sleeping in an unfamiliar bed and anxious about getting your wake-up call. Fortunately, the hotel industry has recognized the need for travelers to have a good night's sleep.

- The Hampton Inn chain (www.hamptoninn.com) based in Memphis, Tennessee poured $80 million into a makeover that included purchasing high-quality mattresses, pillows, comforters, and sheets.

- The Westin (www.starwood.com/westin) offers a comfortable night's rest on its Heavenly Bed.

- Crowne Plaza Hotels and Resorts (www.crowneplaza.com) launched a Sleep Advantage Program that includes comfortable new beds, "Quiet Zone" floors, amenities such as an eye mask and drape clip to block out unwanted light, earplugs, lavender spray, and a sleep CD of relaxation tips and exercises.

When booking your hotel or motel reservation, ask about any "sleep-friendly" rooms that may be available (see also Chapter 3). At the very least, you can request a room away from the nightclub, bar, restaurant, and elevator. If space in your luggage permits, consider packing a familiar object from home that may help make your slumber more peaceful. And if you're really worried about your wake-up call, ask for two.

Stress Factor #8: "Are We There Yet?"

Horror stories about traveling with the kids go something like this: The parents dread traveling with their children. As they pile them into the car or onto the plane, they hope for the best but fear the worst. They wish for soundproof walls between the front and the back seats, and for not having to clean up tons of cracker crumbs just this once. They drive a few extra hours, trying to make it to Aunt Mary's by midnight, and in the meantime they wonder why little Susie is crying so much and why Tommy is hungry again when he just ate a few hours ago. Who wants a trip like this?!

It's not a good idea to start your journey already expecting the worst from your children. But you do need to remember that kids are likely to get bored, tired, upset, and stressed out when they travel, because they are not home, in their regular beds, or going through their regular schedules. So first you should expect this, and then you should plan for it. Bring extra batteries for your son who will fall apart if his videogame stops working. Bring favorite snacks for your daughter who always says she's hungry but only picks at her meals. And consider sticking as closely as possible to some semblance of your home routine—whether it's stopping to rest at a usual naptime or bringing something from home to make the kids more comfortable—especially with little ones or with children who don't adapt well to change.

Food and entertainment are two critical factors in traveling successfully with kids. If you are flying, try to get them a snack or meal before boarding. If a meal will be served on the plane, ask the flight attendant whether the children can be fed first. Inquire whether the airline has any amenities available for kids. British Airways (www.british-airways.com), for example, offers Activity Packs for use at the gate and on the flight, with such diversions as coloring books, crayons, and crossword puzzles.

Whatever your mode of travel, have each child pack his/her own backpack with favorite treats (such as a favorite flavor of gum for plane rides), cards, electronic games, a book, notebook and pencil, portable CD player, and so on. Check out websites like www.momsminivan.com for great travel games. An old favorite is "The Word Game," in which you pick a topic and the children have to name things in that topic without repeating what's already been said—if they get stuck, they have five seconds before they're out. (See also the Resources section in the back of the book.)

An additional strategy is to visit the local dollar store before your trip and pick out a few surprises to give to your children when you hear arguments or those infamous words, "I'm bored." (*Author's note: My rule is that even if the kids haven't complained or argued, they can't resort to saying "I'm bored" until we are at least a fourth of the way through the trip, which forces them to enjoy what they brought for a while before getting one of their trip surprises. —Lisa*)

If you can afford some extra time, don't rush the trip. Remember that kids need breaks to run off pent-up energy, especially when riding in the car. Stop frequently—at least every two to three hours—for a bathroom break to avoid the "Mom, I have to go *now!*" scenario. Rest stops can be miles apart, so have a backup plan; for example, if you have really little ones, consider keeping a portable potty-seat in the trunk. (*Author's note: I traveled with my children after my daughter was potty-trained, but I wasn't sure she would be able to wait for the next rest-stop, so I used Pull-Ups on her for the car ride. It wasn't a step backward in training, and it did help to prevent any potentially messy accidents along the way. —Lisa*)

Your children may want to stay up late when you're all on vacation, but try not to make it night after night, or you may end up spending most of your time consoling a passel of cranky kids—some vacation! If you plan on a late night, consider scheduling an easier morning for the following day. Know what your children are capable of and let them have fun, but if they get overtired and miserable, you won't enjoy yourself either. Of course, if your kids don't need downtime or are okay when they stay up late, that's fine too. It's important to figure out what works for *your* family, and every family is different.

Stress Factor #9: Gridlock

Bumper-to-bumper traffic can make you want to turn the car around and go home. Bring a map so you can find alternative routes around a traffic jam without getting lost! But if you get stuck and it can't be helped, you and your traveling companions can make the best of your unwanted "time out" by keeping little things to do in the car. (Obviously, for most of the following activities, the driver is only to be doing them if the car is not moving. Safety first!)

McStress Relief

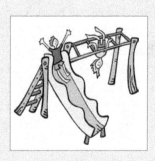

Take advantage of the free play areas offered at many fast-food restaurants such as McDonald's and Burger King. These can be good places—in a pinch—for everyone to stretch their legs and burn off some energy along the road. Meanwhile, the adults can also take their time eating without the little ones getting fidgety at the table.

- Listen to an audiobook or a new CD, or challenge yourself with a language tape.
- Bring a tape recorder to dictate notes about your trip or a to-do list for work or home.
- Do isometric exercises (see the inset Anti-Stress Press on page 71).
- Pick up a few favorite DVDs for the road, so passengers—not the driver—can pop in a movie. (Remember: in some states, it's illegal for the driver to watch a television while driving—and of course, it's a complete lack of common sense for the driver to do so in any state!)
- Daydream.
- Read short pieces in periodicals like *Reader's Digest.*
- Pay bills.
- Check your email with your PDA or laptop.
- Clear your mind by meditating, or by counting backward from fifty.
- Use your cell phone to return calls or make appointments (haircuts, dentist, veterinarian, and the like).
- Keep snacks and drinks handy (not in the trunk) to handle hunger pangs.
- Soothe your car's occupants with the smell of lavender by putting a few drops of the oil on a bandana or other piece of fabric on the front seat.

Traffic is starting to move again? Driver, eyes back on the road. . . .

Stress Factor #10: The Ones You Leave Behind

If you're a frequent business traveler, you're probably keyed up to be back home, but your spouse doesn't even notice—he/she is irritable and tense. What's wrong? Studies have shown that your busy travel schedule may be physically and emotionally affecting your spouse. In fact, stress-related psychological disorders, skin diseases, and intestinal diseases are three times more likely to occur in people whose spouses travel frequently.

"When one partner leaves on business, the whole load of household and family responsibility falls on the spouse remaining at home," says Dr.

Anti-Stress Press

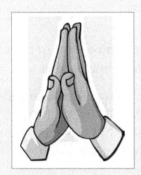

"As you probably know, isometric exercise is when you press your muscles against each other or against a stationary object to build strength," says Kelly James-Enger, certified personal trainer and coauthor of *Small Changes, Big Results: A 12-Week Action Plan to a Better Life* (New York, NY: Clarkson Potter, 2005). She suggests the following easy isometric exercises that you can do in the car:

■ Bring your hands together as if you are praying, press your hands against each other (you'll feel it in your arms and chest) and hold for five seconds, then rest. Start with five repetitions.

■ You can also place one hand over the other with your hands lower (near your lap), one facing up and one down, and press; this uses your arm muscles more.

James-Enger recommends using gridlock time to do a posture check-up too. "Are you slumping? Is your head hanging down? Take a moment and imagine there's a string at the top of your head, pulling you upright. Stretch your shoulders back, tighten your abdominal muscles (imagine sucking your stomach in), and hold the position for five to ten seconds. Don't hold your breath, though; breathe slowly and deeply, and just focus on holding your abs tight. It will strengthen your core and improve your posture."

Tessina. "If the plumbing goes out, or a childhood illness or knotty parenting issue arises, the at-home partner is effectively in the same situation as a single parent. The at-home person often feels as if the traveling partner gets all the perks (hotel room service, social events with business associates, the ability to escape routine), leaving the at-home partner stuck with all the day-to-day problems. This builds resentment and creates power struggles between the partners."

How can couples handle these problems of lengthy or frequent separation? "Stay in touch," advises Dr. Tessina. "The traveling partner needs to make sure the at-home partner feels appreciated, and to be as much a part of decisions made at home as possible." If you are the traveling partner, you can do the following things to make your at-home partner's life easier while you're away:

- Work together as a team.

- Before you leave, make certain he/she has a support network of friends and/or family, and make arrangements for extra help if needed.

- Although mixing business and pleasure doesn't always work, consider making a solo business trip a family affair instead. Taking your children on a business trip may seem like sheer madness, but more and more travelers are creating family time by toting the tots along.

Traveler to Traveler

In order to make my flights more enjoyable, I always bring something with me that I have been dying to read. If a magazine comes in the mail the week before, I save it for the flight, or I buy a book I have long wanted to read. This makes me look forward to the time on the plane.

—Kathy McCabe

A suggestion for a couple traveling together (or for two friends wearing different sizes of clothing) is to split-pack your clothing. Pack half your clothes in the guy's suitcase, and the guy packs half his clothes in the gal's suitcase. Remember to pack matching outfits in each suitcase. This is really thinking ahead in case one of the suitcases never arrives! At least this way, you'll have some clothes for both.

—www.cruisereviews.com

For overseas or long flights, I bring a silk sleeping mask and spray it with lavender oil before I put it on. Lavender is famous for its relaxing properties. With the mask close to my nose, I'm able to inhale the lavender and fall asleep. It feels like a luxurious treat, but it is easy to do.

—Kathy McCabe, *Dream of Italy,*
www.dreamofitaly.com

Try Shiatsu. It will relax you, and if you're tired, it will wake you up. It's pressing on a series of points on your head or neck.

—Jerry V. Teplitz, *Travel Stress,* www.teplitz.com

I've overheard many customers denied service at the rental car desk because their driver's license had just expired. One customer's license had expired at midnight and it was 1:00 A.M. If our plane had arrived on time at 9:00 P.M., he would have been in the clear. Of course, getting back on the plane after the trip would still have presented problems for him. Always check your license before traveling.

—Connie Meyer

I've joined
the frequent-renter club for all the car-
rental agencies, even though I only rent cars about
six to eight times per year. I get to skip the line and
go right to the counter. The time-saving
factor is enormous.

—Connie Meyer

As a national speaker and author, I travel all the time and do a number of things to keep myself stress free. I ease tension by taking kava and drinking Tension Tamer tea. I keep a smile on my face and talk to people to help them feel more at ease. I joke with the people who are searching my luggage. I say prayers as the plane takes off. I take with me special things that ease my mind— small angels I travel with, and books I enjoy. I call people at the airport that I love and connect with them.

—Jill Lublin, *Guerrilla Publicity with Jay Levinson*
(interview, Adams Media Corporation, Avon, MA, 2002)

Already stressed? Place a 5-inch rubber ball under your head and neck and breathe, slowly rolling over the surface of the ball. 'Ball therapy' reduces stress and eases muscle tension. Different-sized kits and various videos are available.

—Elaine Petrone,
stress-reduction expert,
www.elainepetrone.com

To decide what to bring, log on to www.weatherchannel.com for the five-day forecast for your travel destination. Travel lightly with clothes of the same colors to avoid multiple wardrobes. Never take more than one suitcase, since airlines are starting to charge for extra weight.

—Lillian Vernon,
catalog founder,
www.lillianvernon.com

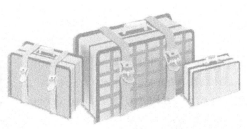

5. Straight-Up Tips for a Healthy Back

YOUR HEAVY CARRY-ON BAG AND POCKETBOOK HANG awkwardly from your shoulder while you desperately try to hold on to that lattè you just bought for the flight and use your other hand to pull your wheeled luggage through the airport. Or worse, you're running late and running through the terminal, perhaps in flip-flops or high-heeled shoes, and you can feel your back wrenching from all the work that you're asking it to do.

You make your flight, but for the next several hours your legs are jammed into an uncomfortable coach seat that doesn't quite accommodate your legs. You try to relax, but there is no comfortable position for your head. After landing, you endure an extra-long car ride to your destination, where you look forward to a restful night after your weary day. Unfortunately, the hotel bed isn't just like the one at home, and you awaken the next day—if you can even sleep—with knotted muscles.

Does this sound like you?

STRAIGHTEN UP AND FLY (OR RIDE) RIGHT

We decided to devote an entire chapter to back care and preventing back pain because we've heard so often from travelers about how their back pain ruined a trip. Many of them didn't have back pain before they traveled, but because of heavy or awkward luggage, long, cramped plane, train, bus, or car rides, and uncomfortable mattresses, their muscles became knotted and started hurting.

"Prolonged sitting can wreak havoc on your body," says Dr. Scott Bautch, immediate past president of the American Chiropractic Association (ACA) Council on Occupational Health. To help prevent problems, Dr. Bautch and the ACA suggest that you treat traveling as an athletic event; that is, warm up before settling into a car or plane seat, and cool down when you reach your destination. Dr. Bautch also recommends taking a brisk walk after a flight, or at regular intervals during long rides, to stretch your hamstring and calf muscles.

There are actually many things you can do for yourself to help prevent back pain, such as packing a lighter suitcase, wearing the proper shoes, enjoying a massage at the terminal's day spa, positioning yourself correctly while you sleep, and bringing the right products to keep your spine aligned and your back pain-free. You may even wish to consult a chiropractor or a physical therapist.

Lugging Your Luggage

Carrying a heavy suitcase by the shoulder-strap can be awkward and stressful on your back muscles; twisting while lifting heavy pieces can be very damaging to the spine; and carrying multiple items puts your back at greater risk for injury. Megan M. Greco, a physical therapist with Physiotherapy Associates in Clarksville, Maryland, instructs travelers to avoid bending and twisting, or reaching and twisting, when moving luggage around. Having treated many patients with shoulder injuries (*Author's note: Including my wife! —Michael*), she also cautions against carrying heavy luggage by its shoulder-strap.

The Travel Goods Association (TGA) advocates a back-friendly approach to luggage. The central idea is to transfer heavy loads away from the shoulders to reduce the strain and impact on the neck, shoulders, and back.

Curious about Chiropractic?

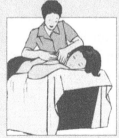

Check out the ACA's website at www.acatoday.com (or call 800-986-4636) to find a doctor of chiropractic near you. You can also obtain additional information about preventing spinal pain and injury, read about effective applications of chiropractic care, and learn about chiropractic education and the history of the profession.

Physician, Heal Thyself: Michael's Story

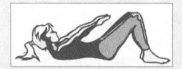 Bonnie Schulman of Mount Washington Physical Therapy in Baltimore, Maryland suggests that you can best serve your back by keeping it in shape on a routine basis—and I can vouch for that. Physical therapy (PT) helped me so much that I was able to cancel my back surgery twenty-four hours before I was scheduled to be wheeled into the operating room.

My morning routine now involves several PT exercises that help keep the spine flexible and strengthen the abdominal muscles, as follows:

- Lying on your back, hug your knees one at a time by wrapping both your arms around the knee, nice and slowly.

- Lying on your back with your knees bent and the soles of your feet on the floor, lift your head and shoulders slightly off the floor while drawing your abdominal muscles toward your spine; hold that position for five or six seconds, then relax, and repeat.

- In the quadruped position (on your hands and knees), do the "Cat and Camel" by alternately rounding your back up with your head hanging down and then arching your back with your head gently lifted up, holding each position for several seconds.

Note: Do not attempt these or other physical therapy exercises without evaluation and proper instruction by a physical therapist.

"New ergonomic designs redistribute the weight of the bag, so transporting it is less taxing on the traveler," says TGA president Michele Marini Pittenger. "On luggage, wheeled systems are better balanced, and handles and shoulder-straps on garment bags, backpacks, and business cases are more comfortably padded."

Protecting your back doesn't only mean packing lightly and using the right luggage, but also learning how to use your back muscles correctly to lift your suitcase. "Remember to use proper body mechanics when putting the luggage in the trunk of the car," says Dr. Ralph Rashbaum, an orthopedic surgeon at the Texas Back Institute. "Brace your knees against the bumper for added support. Do not try to place luggage to the back of the trunk; put a piece of cardboard down first so you can easily push it to the back of the trunk."

Here are additional luggage-handling tips from the Texas Back Institute (www.texasback.com).

- Pack light. Don't stuff so many items into a bag or suitcase that it's almost impossible to lift. Consider dividing heavy items between several bags. (You may also want to consider luggage-free traveling; see Chapter 4.)

- Rent a cart at the airport to alleviate any strain on your back.

- When lifting something heavy, never bend at the waist to pick it up! Always use the power of your thighs, because those muscles are very resistant to strain. Put one knee on the ground, pull the object up on your thigh close to your body, and then stand up.

- Invest in a suitcase with wheels and a handle so you can pull your luggage behind you instead of carrying it in your arms.

Take Your Back for a Joy Ride

The ACA (www.aca.com) gives the following several tips for a pain-free back while driving:

- Adjust the seat so you are as close to the steering wheel as comfortably possible. Your knees should be slightly higher than your hips. Place four fingers behind the back of your thigh close to your knee; if you cannot easily slide your fingers in and out of that space, you need to readjust your seat.

- Consider a back support. Using a support behind your back may reduce the risk of low-back strain, pain, or injury. The widest part of the support should be between the bottom of your ribcage and your waistline. (*Author's note: "Belt-line" might be a better description. Lumbar support is the objective. —Michael*)

- Exercise your legs while driving to reduce the risk of any swelling, fatigue, or discomfort. Spread your toes out as wide as you can, and count to ten. Count to five while you tighten your calf muscles, then your thigh muscles, and then your gluteal muscles. Roll your shoulders forward and back—making sure to keep your hands on the steering wheel and your eyes on the road!

- To minimize arm and hand tension while driving, hold the steering wheel at the clock-face positions of 3:00 and 7:00, and periodically switch your hand placement to the positions of 10:00 and 5:00.

- Do not grip the steering wheel. Instead, tighten and loosen your grasp to improve hand circulation and decrease muscle fatigue in the arms, wrists, and hands.

Products to Protect and Pamper Your Back

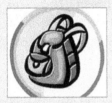 ■ The TGA mentioned previously is a national trade association that represents the manufacturers, distributors, and retailers of luggage, leather goods, computer cases, handbags, and other products for people who travel (visit www.travel-goods. org).

■ The HoMedics Contact Therapy Back Massaging Cushion is a heated, programmable back massager that has three different massage styles and ten pressure points. It includes a car adaptor that plugs into the car lighter (www.homedics.com).

■ The Moller Back Support System (www.mollersupport.com), clinically tested by neurologists at the METS Clinic in San Rafael, California, is the only back support approved by a major airline for use in the cockpit and in flight-training simulators.

■ Travelon has a good selection of travel accessories, including the Soft-Eze Comfort Pillow and the Sensor-Touch Comfort Pillow (www.travelon bags.com or 800-537-5544).

■ Check out the website www.travelpro.com for innovative luggage designed for traveling professionals.

■ The Samsonite Chiropak Backpack is endorsed by the ACA and ergonomically designed to reduce muscle fatigue and stress on the spine (at Samsonite locations nationwide and www.samsonitecompanystores.com).

■ Visit the website www.healthyback.com for more supplies to maintain a healthy back.

- While always being careful to keep your eyes on the road, vary your focal point while driving to reduce the risk of eye fatigue and tension headaches.

- Take rest breaks. Never underestimate the potential consequences of fatigue to yourself, your passengers, and other drivers.

Back Pain Relief for Travelers

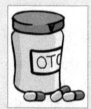

Over-the-counter medications such as aspirin, ibuprofen, or acetaminophen may provide temporary relief, or perhaps you require something stronger. Make sure to discuss any existing back problems with your physician before you leave, so you'll know what medication is best and can obtain any necessary prescriptions.

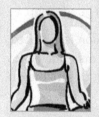

Practice yoga. Wendy Brenner's intriguing article "Traveling with a Bad Back" (*Travel and Leisure* online, www.travelandleisure.com, October 1997; excerpted with permission) describes her unorthodox method of preventing midair back pain—it gets her a few stares, but she doesn't care. "One-Minute Mystery: Returning from a business trip, on layover in some American airport, you notice a young woman in cowboy boots attempting to hide behind a bank of pay phones. Then she shuts her eyes and squats deeply in the position used by Hindu gods with multiple pairs of arms . . . On the plane, it turns out she is your seatmate. You never get up the nerve to ask what she was doing earlier . . . Although it's a seventy-minute flight, the woman makes four trips to the back of the plane, each time toting two of those Chiclet-sized airline pillows and what appears to be an orange golf ball . . . the answer won't surprise anyone who suffers from chronic back problems. The woman was me, the squat is a 'hatha yoga' posture, and it breaks up muscle spasms." (Have you seen Wendy on *your* flight?)

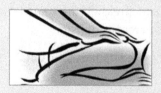

Plan time to get a massage at a local spa, at your hotel, or even at the airport. Massage is a great way to prevent or relieve those travel-related kinks.

The ACA recommends the following procedures to protect your back when traveling by airplane:

- Stand up straight and feel the normal "s"-curve of your spine. Then use rolled up pillows or blankets to maintain that curve when you sit in your seat. Tuck a pillow behind your back just above the belt-line, and lay another pillow across the gap between your neck and the headrest. If the seat is hollowed from wear, use folded blankets to raise your buttocks a little.

- Check all bags that are heavier than 15 to 20 percent of your body weight. Overhead lifting of any significant amount of weight should be avoided to reduce the risk of pain in the lower back or neck. While lifting your bags, stand right in front of the overhead compartment so the spine is not rotated. Do not turn or twist your head and neck in the process.

> **"The Art and Science of Travelling Light"**
>
> Visit the website www.onebag.com for numerous how-to suggestions on traveling with a single bag.

- When stowing belongings under the seat, do not force the object with an awkward motion using your legs, feet, or arms, as this may cause muscle strain or spasms in the upper thighs and lower back muscles. Instead, sit in your seat first, and using your hands and feet, gently guide your bags under the seat directly in front of you.

- While seated, vary your position occasionally to improve circulation and avoid leg cramps. Massage legs and calves. Bring your legs in and move your knees up and down. Prop your legs up on a book or a bag under your seat.

- Do not sit directly under the air controls. The draft can increase tension in your neck and shoulder muscles.

Put Your Best Foot Forward

When you travel, your feet can take a beating, which can throw your back out of whack. Save the high-heeled pumps for your nice dinner out, keep the flip-flops for the beach, and wear a pair of good, flat walking shoes (with a 1-inch heel or lower). Never bring a brand-new pair of shoes or sneakers on a trip! If you're going to need new shoes for the trip, buy them at least a month ahead of time and wear them frequently to break them in (see also Chapter 6).

When purchasing your shoes, remember that all feet differ and that a proper fit is definitely not based on appearance. According to podiatrist James Adleberg, D.P.M., body weight, foot structure, arch, width, and special problems like tendonitis, shin splints, and bursitis must all be taken into consideration. Many sneakers are made with comfortably padded heels to provide support and stability for the legs and feet. Walking shoes should also support the heel at a higher level than the rest of the foot and maintain ample room in the toe-box.

Ergonomic Travel and Lodging

Ergonomics, defined in *Dorland's Medical Dictionary* as "the science relating to humans and their work, embodying the anatomic, physiologic, psychologic, and mechanical principles affecting the efficient use of human energy," is another important consideration for the traveler, both in transit and at rest. Some airlines have changed their seat designs to eliminate joint pressure and reduce musculoskeletal problems in passengers, especially on long flights.

Many hotels have also considered ergonomically correct seats, mattresses, and workstations in their room and decor designs. When you make your reservation, remember that mattresses, pillows, and other accessories cannot always be individualized to suit your particular needs, but do ask to have a firm mattress if possible. When it's time for some shut-eye, the best way to sleep (ergonomically speaking) is on your side with your knees bent. Put a pillow under your head to support your neck and another one between your knees. If you must sleep on your back, put pillows under your knees and a small pillow under your lower back. Don't sleep on your stomach unless you put a pillow under your hips.

Back Care for the Kids, Too

It's important to protect your children's spines and back muscles from the rigors of travel as well. Make sure they have adequate footwear, and keep a watchful eye on their backpacks. It's great for kids to have their own special bag of toys and treats for the journey, but it shouldn't be too big or too heavy for them to carry comfortably. And to safeguard your little tyke in transit, here are several important car-seat tips from the ACA (www.acatoday.com).

- Always use a car seat in a car when traveling with children under the age of four and weighing less than 40 pounds.

- Make sure the car seat is appropriate for the age and size of the child. A newborn infant requires a different seat than a three-year-old toddler does.

- Car seats for infants should always face the rear. In this position, the force and impact of a crash will be spread more evenly along the back and shoulders, providing more protection for the neck.

- Car seats should always be placed in the back seat of the car, ideally in the center of the back seat (to avoid potential impact with the front seats or passengers in the event of a collision). This is especially important in cars equipped with airbags. If an airbag is deployed, the force could seriously injure or kill a child or infant placed in the front seat.

- Make sure the car seat is properly secured to the seat of the vehicle and is placed at a 45-degree angle to support the head of the infant or child.

- Ask your airline for their policy on child car-seat safety. Car seats for infants and toddlers provide added resistance to turbulent skies, and are safer than the lap of a parent in the event of an accident.

Traveler to Traveler

I had a sprained shoulder several years ago and still suffer from pain in my right shoulder and my back, across the shoulder blades. It can become quite extreme at times, and plane travel exacerbates it. If I know I'm going to be taking a trip, I try to work on my shoulder muscles for the week preceding the travel—doing stretching exercises, getting massages, applying heat/ice. I also use ThermaCare patches, thin, self-adhesive patches that generate low heat when applied to the skin. You can wear them under clothing and the heat keeps the muscle relaxed. I also take those single-use, crunch-up cold packs for quick relief of serious pain. Once I was traveling to Hawaii (long plane ride) on business. I was going to have an intense, active schedule and long days once I got there. I was worried I would arrive in pain, so I went two days early and booked a room at a nice resort with a spa so I could rest, recover and—if necessary—book a massage and sit in the hot tub.

—freelance writer Hilda J. Brucker

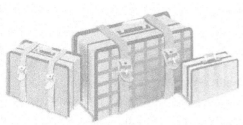

6. Healthy Body

WE ALL KNOW THAT EATING RIGHT AND EXERCISING are two main staples of a healthful lifestyle. When you're traveling, however, finding healthful food and fitting in your regular exercise routine can be arduous tasks—unless you look into your options beforehand.

You can always use the hotel gym or stroll around the property, of course, but did you know you might also be able to take your hometown gym membership on the road, or even work out at the airport? At your destination, you can hike on nearby paths or take a city walking tour. If you pack the right stuff, maybe you can enjoy a swim, or exercise in the privacy of your room. And when you're looking for that next healthful meal, many restaurant menus now offer myriad low-carbohydrate or vegetarian options, or meals with "points" for people using the Weight Watchers' system (see Chapter 7 for much more information about eating). Even the fast-food joints feature salads nowadays!

This chapter and the next are devoted to showing you how to stay fit when you're traveling. Of course that doesn't mean you can't enjoy yourself, eat a few rich, hearty meals, and skip a workout or two. After all, it's a vacation! But studies show that keeping to a regular fitness routine and eating carefully can help you reduce your chances of illness and prevent stress on your trip.

KEEP IT SIMPLE AND DO YOUR BEST

In "A Traveler's Workout Guide" (*The Physician and Sportsmedicine* Vol. 26 [1998]), Dr. Bryant Stamford suggests keeping expectations realistic about workouts during travel. "Jaunts out of town can . . . leave your fitness pro-

Your Personal Fitness Monitor

BalanceLog makes it easy to log and track your eating and exercise habits on a Palm OS PDA or a Windows PC, even when traveling. BalanceLog (available at www.healthetech. com) provides the nutritional content of 3,000 foods and the value of 300 exercises, and you can add favorite foods and menus to further customize the database. Each user's nutrition profile includes daily targets for calories, protein, carbohydrates, fats, dietary cholesterol, sodium, fiber, and sugar.

gram bankrupt. Travel, it seems, was designed to disrupt your daily routine, sleep pattern, and diet. The result can be stress and fatigue that dampen your desire to exercise. In addition, lack of facilities and nonstop meetings can rob you of opportunities to work out."

But that doesn't mean you should give up on the idea entirely. Stamford writes, "If you are well rested and blessed with sufficient facilities and time, go for it. For some travelers, hotel health clubs and free evenings provide ideal opportunities to boost their fitness. If they also strive to eat healthfully by focusing on wise food selections, they can even come back home a bit healthier than when they left."

Of the many tips in this chapter, this one is the most important: don't overwhelm yourself. Don't try to have the perfect workout or schedule a bunch of different activities. Instead, pick a favorite (or two)—whether it's walking, in-room exercise to videos, swimming, tennis, or a jog—and make it a point to do it regularly. How long should you work out? Aim for at least thirty minutes of moderate activity each day, or three ten-minute sessions throughout the course of the day. (If you are traveling to a high altitude, however, remember to take it easy and avoid overexerting yourself for a few days after reaching your destination; see Chapter 2.)

Traveling Gyms

Don't leave home without it . . . your gym membership, that is! Before your trip, contact your fitness company's home office or visit its website for a directory of the company's clubs or programs at various destinations, and check your contract for travel benefits eligibility.

At some clubs, membership with travel privileges costs more than a standard membership. For example, Bally Total Fitness (www.ballyfitness.

com) has a higher-priced membership option that allows frequent travelers to use any of Bally's 400 centers within twenty-eight states and Canada. Crunch Fitness (www.crunch.com) offers a Passport Membership for an additional $100 that permits the use of Crunch clubs nationwide. LA Fitness (www.lafitness.com) offers a higher-rate Platinum Membership valid at all LA Fitness clubs in all states; this also includes two guest privileges per visit, which can be beneficial if you are meeting or traveling with a business associate.

Some fitness facilities, however, grant free travel privileges. Lady of America (www.ladyofamerica.com) honors all its memberships throughout the country at no additional charge and without any limitations on use. Curves (www.curvesinternational.com) provides a Travel Pass that allows members to use any other Curves facility. Most YMCAs (visit www.ymca.net) honor memberships in any Y. Several clubs also honor memberships worldwide with no extra fee but with certain restrictions. World Gym International (www.worldgym.com) and Gold's Gym (www.golds gym.com) offer members travel cards to use at a branch at least fifty miles outside their hometown at no additional charge, for no more than fourteen days annually per gym.

If your club isn't a chain with nationwide facilities, don't despair. The International Health, Racquet, and Sportsclub Association (IHRSA;

Opportunistic Exercising

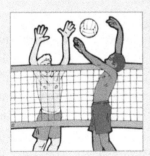

You aren't obligated to stay in your room, and your exercise needn't be limited to a fixed workout routine or a standard fitness club. Be creative in your activities, and use whatever is around you as you go. Build exercise into a jam-packed trip schedule by fast-walking through the airport and using the stairs at your hotel. Instead of spending all your free time lying by the pool, jump in and do some water-aerobics or water-jogging. Have fun biking, water-skiing, walking along the water, or playing beach volleyball. Looking for souvenirs? Put in a few brisk laps at the local mall, then slow down and reward yourself.

Take Your Swimming Program on the Road

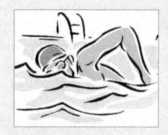

United States Masters Swimming (USMS) is a national, nonprofit corporation that provides organized workouts, competitions, clinics, and workshops for adult swimmers age eighteen and over (fitness, triathlete, competitive, and noncompetitive), with programs at 500 clubs in fifty-three regions throughout the United States. *The Swimmers Guide Online* at the USMS website (www.usms.org; click on the "Places to Swim" tab) lists 12,369 swimming facilities with 13,155 full-sized, year-round swimming pools in 7,150 cities and towns in the nation and in 129 foreign countries.

www.ihrsa.org or cms.ihrsa.org) established a Passport Program allowing members of more than 3,600 IHRSA-affiliated gyms worldwide the privilege of working out in clubs that are not usually open to travelers, either for free or at a substantially discounted rate. For example, if your fitness facility in Los Angeles is an IHRSA-affiliated gym, you can request a Passport Program identification card, have it stamped and signed, and use the Boston Racquet Club when you travel there. Restrictions state that your home club must be at least fifty miles from the club you are visiting. To find participating clubs, visit the website www.healthclubs.com.

Flying Gyms?

No need to dread that four-hour layover—it's a perfect opportunity to utilize the airport's fitness center! At McCarran Airport in Las Vegas, 24-Hour Fitness offers packages for travelers who bring their own workout clothes and gear ($15 for facilities and towel), and can also provide gear for use at the center. The Westin Detroit Metropolitan Airport Hotel is another twenty-four-hour exercise center with cardio equipment, an indoor pool, and a whirlpool. Day passes (from $8) are available at Chicago O'Hare International Airport's Hilton Hotel Athletic Club, the Fairmont Vancouver Airport Hotel, and the Miami International Airport Hotel. (See also Chapter 4.)

You may even be able to fit in some in-flight exercise. Last year, JetBlue teamed up with Crunch Fitness and launched a Flying Pilates program "to bring fitness and inner peace to the skies" with a seat-pocket card suggesting four Pilates moves to "de-stress" while seated. For an $8 fee, Song Airlines (Delta Airlines) offers passengers an elastic band, a squeezable ball, and a how-to manual designed by star gym-owner David Barton to guide the seated workout.

A ROOM WITH A VIEW... AND A TREADMILL

If you don't want to make a club commitment, or if there isn't a convenient fitness chain at home, check out the hotels, motels, and bed-and-breakfasts at your destination. Some will loan equipment or even provide in-room instruction to help you stay on track with your workout regimen. The certified fitness concierges at the Affinia DuMont and Dumont Plaza Suites hotels in New York City (www.affinia.com) and Don Shula's Hotel in Miami Lakes, Florida (www.donshulahotel.com) arrange personal training appointments, find jogging trails, and lead fitness workshops.

If you are hoping to use the hotel gym, it's important to be informed and alert. According to Suzanne Schlosberg (author of *Fitness for Travelers: The Ultimate Workout Guide for the Road*, Boston, MA: Houghton Mifflin, 2002), exercise amenities at hotels vary widely: "Many of the weight machines are of high quality, while others have deteriorating cables, torn seat padding, and substandard engineering that could end up separating you from your shoulder." Schlosberg suggests asking specific questions about the gym equipment when booking your reservation, and even touring the facility before paying for the room. "At mid-priced establishments you might find one treadmill and a small array of dumbbells, or none at all," she says.

Many hotels—even moderately priced chains—have now upgraded their fitness facilities to include state-of-the-art equipment, racquetball courts, classes, trainers, and more. Stillwater Spa Suites guests of the Hyatt Regency Lake Tahoe Resort, Spa, and Casino (www.hyatt.com) can enjoy in-room Life Fitness Cycles. Guests at the Fairmont Turnberry Isle Resort and Club in Florida (www.fairmont.com) can rent rooms equipped with treadmills and Shiatsu massage chairs. Rental equipment at the Four Seasons in New York City (www.fourseasons.com) includes treadmills, bikes, and Stairmasters (upward of $150 per day).

To help "decompress" your body, book a room at one of the Kimpton Hotels (www.kimptonhotels.com), which feature a continuous in-room yoga television channel and a complimentary "yoga basket" with a mat, block, and strap for all guests. Boston's Beacon XV (www.xvbeacon.com) offers in-room yoga (a tad pricey, but what a treat). The Four Seasons, the Hilton (www.hilton.com), and several other hotels offer affordable (sometimes free) packages that include clothing, shoes, weights, resistance bands, yoga mat, and exercise videos.

Consider the variety of exercise options available to travelers when you're choosing where to stay, and inquire about the health club amenities on site or nearby when you make your reservation (if the reservationist doesn't know, ask to speak to the hotel concierge). Hotels and motels often partner with area gyms to offer free or low-cost passes to hotel guests. Here are several examples:

- The Fitzpatrick Grand Central and Manhattan Hotels in New York City (www.fitzpatrickhotels.com) offer complimentary memberships to the Excelsior Athletic Club and the New York Sports Club, both within walking distance.

A Fitness Vacation

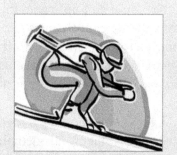

"Make your next vacation a fitness theme. Skiing and backpacking are both activities that get you outside and get your heart pumping. Check with local environmental organizations, recreation clubs, or university programs to see what group vacations they offer. Kayaking, trekking, and scuba vacations are all very popular, and will incorporate fitness, fun, and adventure. Just make sure you plan ahead so that you are in the proper shape, and properly trained, to take on these activities. So hiking the Himalayas isn't your thing. Even if you choose to relax at a resort or on a tropical beach, you're still steps from a good workout. Hit the pool or the ocean for a swim, walk the golf course instead of renting a cart, or challenge your travel partner to a jog down the beach (save the strolling for sunset)."

—The American Council on Exercise, www.acefitness.org

- Southmoreland Bed and Breakfast in Kansas City, Missouri (www.southmoreland.com) has arrangements with two local fitness centers including the indoor pool and exercise facility at nearby St. Luke's Hospital.

- Best Suites in Rockford, Illinois (www.qsrockford.com) offers free passes to the neighboring Bally Total Fitness club.

- Local fitness facilities give guests of the Fairmont Hotels in Vancouver, Chicago, Santa Monica, and New Orleans (www.fairmont.com) a low-cost daily rate (access is free for members of the hotel's President's Club).

- Guests of the Holiday Inn Express in Hendersonville, Tennessee (www.ichotelsgroup.com) can use the next-door YMCA free of charge.

Portable Exercise Gear

Of course you can't take it all, but some exercise equipment does pack easily:

- Jump rope (see the Traveler to Traveler tip on page 93).

- Resistance bands or tubing—hook them to a doorknob or other handle to perform a variety of exercises that won't place undue stress on your joints.

- Pedometer.

- Travel weights—Aquabells, for example, provide up to 16 pounds of resistance per dumbbell when filled with water at your destination, but weigh less than 26 ounces when empty and are compact enough to fit in a briefcase (a set of two 13-inch bars with cushioned grip handles and eight fillable weights at www.aquabells.com/specs.html for $49.95; ankle weights are also available).

Exercise videos or DVDs are terrific for working out on your own schedule in the privacy of your room. Try Denise Austin's exercise videos, which offer target workouts for a flatter stomach, slimmer waistline, and stronger lower back; for example, *Get Fit Fast: Abs*, a forty-minute video broken down into three levels of workouts, and *The Ultimate Fat Burner*, thirty-five minutes of fat burning and toning divided into seven high-intensity sections of aerobic exercise and weight training (available at www.deniseaustin.com).

The right sneakers, of course, are a vital part of most exercise efforts. Heed the following advice:

- Buy running or walking shoes in the evening, when your feet are slightly swollen.

- To ensure a proper fit, wear socks, try on more than one size of the same shoe, and make sure you have a finger-width space between your longest toe and the shoe tip.

- Do not sacrifice comfort to buy a cheaper pair.

- Do not bring a brand-new pair on your trip; instead, wear them regularly at least a week or two before you leave. Remember, however, that the best footwear does not need much "breaking in." (See also Put Your Best Foot Forward on page 81.)

Finally, don't forget to pack comfortable, breathable workout clothes and any exercise accessories you may require: weight-lifting gloves, swimming gear (suit, goggles, earplugs, and nose plug), sports bra, jock strap, and the like.

Hit the Net

And we don't mean the tennis court (although that may also be an option). Today's traveler can find numerous fitness opportunities, weight-management tips, and even a personal trainer online. Great fitness websites include www.efit.com, which offers healthful-living tools like a calorie counter, body mass index, message boards, and more, and www.fitnesszone.com, which helps you find an exercise facility in its listing of 13,000 gyms and health clubs. (See also the Resources section in the back of the book.)

Unlike most travel databases, Fit for Business (www.fitforbusiness. com) isn't paid by the hotels and gyms it describes—the only way to get listed on this website is to have a great facility. The database tells you what you can expect in both first-class fitness and business amenities, from the dumbbells and type of squash court to the availability of two-line telephone hook-ups. The Fit for Business site also offers Achieve, a benefit package for athletic frequent travelers, who enjoy waived or reduced admission fees at many hotel-associated athletic clubs as well as reduced rates for club services such as personal training, court time, and massage. Sweatime, an online scheduling service for many of these clubs, enables Achieve members to check group exercise times, make appointments, and find playing partners at the clubs they visit.

Traveling with a personal trainer is not only for the rich and famous. The website www.myfitnessexpert.com, partnered with the American College of Sports Medicine, assigns you a real trainer who answers your emails, sets up your programs based on your available equipment, sends you reminders, and checks on your progress. If you sign up for one-year service, the fee is only $19.99 per month—not bad! (*Author's note: I tried the site and was quite impressed with the trainer's diligence in asking for medical background information and not assigning a program unless those questions were answered. —Lisa*)

 Traveler to Traveler

After watching my daughter in the Jump Rope for Heart Program from the American Heart Association, I took one of her jump-ropes and left it in my suitcase. Even if the hotel doesn't have a fitness center, there is always a corner of the parking lot or sidewalk near the pool that I can use. It is safer than jogging through neighborhoods I don't know or along the busy roads that usually surround hotels. After thirty minutes of jumping, some stretching, push-ups, and sit-ups, one has a great, 'heart-healthy,' and cheap workout. Don't plan on jumping rope in your room unless you are on the first floor—I found the people below you aren't very appreciative of your exercising above them.

—Traveling fitness buff Tad Druart

If the hotel doesn't have a workout room, I'll run stairs and skip rope, or if there is no access to stairs, I'll go into the parking lot and skip rope. (Yes, I get weird looks, but no one bothers me!!)

—Melyssa St. Michael, *Becoming a Personal Trainer for Dummies* (Hoboken, NJ: Wiley Publishing, Inc., 2004; www.dummies.com)

My body is the best piece of equipment I have! I get a great workout from push-ups, lunges, incline push-ups, squats, crunches, every possible bodyweight movement I can think of I do—fast!—to keep my heart rate up and give myself a challenging workout. Desk chairs are great (the ones without wheels) in the hotel room because you can perform step-ups on them, do dips off of them, put your feet on them and do decline push-ups.

—Melyssa St. Michael

Keep it fun! Incorporate exercise into your fun activities without thinking 'workout.' If you're lounging by the pool or cruising the Caribbean, jump in the pool every thirty minutes or so. Don't just stand there sipping on that daiquiri— jog in place, do standing leg-lifts, swim, or hold on to the wall and kick your heart out!

—Jyl Steinback, www.AmericasHealthiestMom.com

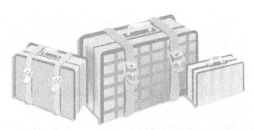

7. Healthy Eating

D O THESE SOUND FAMILIAR? "I can eat that now, I'm on vacation!" or "I'll worry about my weight when I get back." Traveling used to be the perfect excuse to go off your diet and indulge your appetite—whether for rich French pastries, down-home Southern cooking, or a sumptuous Italian spread. After all, who wanted to count calories when you were supposed to be having fun? And traveling on business was the perfect opportunity to explore a new eatery and treat a potential client to a rich, satisfying meal.

It was also hard to resist the fast-food joints lining the nation's highways and airport terminals. The greasy burger that seemed to call your name was bound to be tastier than airplane food. With healthful options few and far between, experts advised travelers to pack nutritious sandwiches and salads. But get real—fries and donuts were much easier and faster to eat one-handed *en route*!

TIMES HAVE CHANGED

Weight Watchers, Jenny Craig, South Beach, or Atkins—these days, who isn't on some sort of weight-loss regimen or healthy eating plan? Although you may want to enjoy some carefree feasting or explore a new cuisine while you're away, you don't want to worry about those extra pounds when you come home. Happily, the hospitality industry has taken notice. Many restaurants and hotels now offer low-carbohydrate menus. Fast-food restaurants feature fruit, yogurt parfaits, and more (and tastier) salad choices. Cruise lines still beckon vacationers to all-you-can-eat buffets supplemented by round-the-clock snacks, but now you'll find lighter fare and more healthful selections.

Breakfast Does a Body Good

"You can absolutely eat healthy while traveling," says Rachel Brandeis, a registered dietician in Atlanta, Georgia, and a spokesperson for the American Dietetic Association (www.eatright.org). "It just takes a little planning and mindfulness."

First, Brandeis suggests to decide daily what meal you want to indulge on, and then plan the rest of the day's eating around it. "For example, if you are going out for three meals that day and you know you're having a blow-out dinner, keep your other two meals healthy. Make the choice to stay on your healthy eating plan or diet."

Second, emphasize healthful breakfasts on your trip. "If you're going to indulge at the breakfast buffets, you can take in 1,000 calories before you even start your day," says Brandeis. "You can also feel sluggish because you have a large amount of food to digest, especially if you choose the fattening foods such as sausage, bacon, waffles, and pastries." Skip the all-you-can-eat smorgasbord and pass on the assorted pastries with the continental breakfast. Instead, choose lighter fare such as whole-grain cereal or oatmeal with skim milk, fruit and yogurt, or an egg with lightly buttered toast. Studies show that if you start your day with the proper fuel, you're also less likely to overindulge on high-calorie, fattening foods for the rest of the day.

Coffee, Tea—or a $10 Meal?

If you haven't flown in quite some time, it may surprise you to learn that many United States flights do not serve free meals anymore. Most domestic airlines that do serve meals, including Northwest, U.S. Airways, Midwest, United, American, America West, and Funjet, require that passengers pay for their food on board. (On some flights, only cash is accepted, so be prepared, because you don't want to be stuck without something to eat.)

Travel writer Sophia Dembling hasn't purchased any of the new buy-on-board airplane meals just yet. "I am perfectly happy to buy plane food, but it would have to be edible," says the author of *The Yankee Chick's Survival Guide to Texas* (www.yankeechick.com). To accommodate the palates of travelers like Dembling, some airline catering companies have secured licensing agreements with recognizable restaurants such as Einstein Brothers, Hard Rock Café, TGI Friday's, and Wolfgang Puck to spice up their menus with a wider variety of more delectable fare. Delectable doesn't necessarily mean healthful, of course, but that all depends on what you order.

Delta's low-fare carrier, Song, for example, has added gourmet and organic selections including yogurt, sushi, and a variety of salads.

Be sure to bring along something healthful to eat, in case the plane or train food isn't to your liking. "Don't ever get on the plane without food and snacks, whether it's peanut butter crackers, energy bars, or single-serving canned fruit," Brandeis advises. You can also find a deli in the terminal and buy a turkey, roast beef, or ham sandwich. "Stay away from fattening or salty snack foods," she says. "But if that's all there is to choose from, then a package of peanuts will give you a longer-lasting fullness than a snack mix."

On the Road Again

When the Herrin family travels by car in Europe, they make a point of avoiding restaurants. "Our three kids (ages four, eight, and ten) would all want to order something different but then eat only a third of it," says mom Jennifer Herrin. "And I'm too cheap to waste money that way! So we always travel with a picnic backpack and ice-chest and then look for a grocery store in a little town. In Europe as in the States, many groceries have fresh pre-made sandwiches and salads—and to me, the stuff in the higher-end groceries is often better than restaurant food. Browsing the aisles and trying new products has actually become one of our favorite things to do when traveling."

Eating healthfully *en route* is probably easiest to do when traveling by car or RV; like Herrin, you can pack delicious, nutritious snacks or picnic baskets and ignore the temptations of roadside restaurants and fast-food stands. But if you do want to stop and eat, pick light choices like salads, fruit, yogurt, or sandwiches. You can easily find out about the eating establishments on your route with a little Internet research before you go. Try the website www.healthyhighways.com by Nikki and David Goldbeck, authors of *Healthy Highways: The Traveler's Guide to Healthy Eating*. These food-and-travel gurus show you how to avoid fast-food pitfalls and make informed choices about where to dine, pick up a healthful snack, or restock your cooler. State maps and local directions guide you to 1,900 healthy eateries and natural food stores throughout the United States.

Slim Pickings

If you arrive at your destination famished and exhausted, you'll probably just settle for whatever is around, be it the hotel buffet, an unfamiliar local restaurant, or the coffee shop down the block. Author Joan Price (www.joanprice.com) has some suggestions on proactively preventing such a situation: "Long before you're tired and hungry, investigate where you can get healthy meals. Before you leave home, get recommendations from friends, read magazine reviews, and do a Web search for restaurants in that city. Once you get to the new city, peruse the Yellow Pages restaurant ads. Ask the concierge. Then phone the restaurants that end up on your list and make sure they offer foods you like."

If you get stuck in a restaurant of someone else's choosing, you don't have to make your best guess from the menu; instead, say to the waitperson, "I have medical reasons for needing to eat a heart-healthy, low-fat diet." (After all, who could deny that *everyone* has medical reasons for eat-

Weight-Management Programs

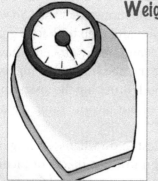

Perhaps you are involved in a weight-management program. Obviously you can't travel with the program's food packed in your suitcase, so what can you do? Take your membership with you instead:

- A Jenny Craig membership can be used at any participating center for no additional cost. Log on to the website www.jennycraig. com and do a zip-code search for centers at or near your travel destination, where you can purchase food items, products, meet with a consultant—in short, do everything you would typically do at your home center.

- Don't worry about missing a Weight Watchers meeting, even when you travel internationally, as Weight Watchers operates eighteen sites in fifteen countries. Visit www.weightwatchers.com and use the free Meeting Finder resource (you can enter the zip code of your next port-of-call for a list of nearby meetings). And at the local Applebee's restaurant, you will find menu selections based on Weight Watchers' points.

- If you're following the Atkins diet, check out the website www.atkinsdiet.meetup.com before you hit the road, to see a list of meetings in more than 650 cities worldwide.

ing a heart-healthy diet?) Just ask before you order, and many restaurants will be happy to prepare something that meets your needs even if it's not on the menu.

The Low-Carb Craze

With more than 35 million Americans counting carbohydrates, many hotels, resorts, cruise lines, and restaurants are now catering to low-carb dieters. Sheraton Hotels and Resorts (www.starwood.com/sheraton, or 888-625-5144), for example, has introduced Lo-Carb Lifestyle by Sheraton in more than 200 hotels worldwide. Lo-Carb Lifestyle features more than fifteen menu items, most containing fewer than five net carbohydrates, to cover all three meals, dessert, snacks, and cocktail nibbles. The program even extends to the iconic hotel treat you'll find on your pillow: a new, sinfully delicious chocolate mint with less than one net carb!

Holiday Inn Hotels and Resorts (www.ichotelsgroup.com), Hyatt (www.hyatt.com), Loews (www.loewshotels.com), Radisson (www.radisson.com), Embassy Suites (www.embassysuites.com), and the Marriott Hotels (www.marriott.com) have all added low-carb options to their menus. Or you can forgo the hotel restaurant and dine at other eateries that have added low-carb options, including Ruby Tuesdays, TGI Fridays, Village Inn, Subway, and Blimpie.

Eatin' and Cruisin'

When travelers decide on a cruise, they're thinking of sun, fun, and food—and lots of it. With three meals and endless snacks and desserts offered each day (and into the night), it's important for cruise passengers to be careful about their food choices. But it's hard to pass up an incredible all-you-can-eat extravaganza—and for some people, the food is one of the best parts of a cruise! If that sounds like you, try these tips for better eating at sea:

- Stay with routine. Eat three healthy meals and a few light snacks. Don't pile on the food at midnight, even if you plan on dancing the night away.

- Don't feel obligated to sit down at every meal. For example, instead of parking yourself next to the platters of pancakes and sausage, grab some yogurt and fruit for breakfast and head to the deck to watch the sunrise.

- Stroll by the dining room earlier in the day to check out the menu. You'll have time to ponder your selection ahead of time without being overwhelmed by temptation at the table; or, you'll see a treat that you *must* have later, and you can plan accordingly for the day.

- Split an entrée with a friend instead of eating the oversized portions.

- Watch what you drink, especially liquor, and try to drink as much bottled water as possible.

Consider booking your trip with one of the several cruise lines making a concerted effort to help their guests maintain an all-around healthful lifestyle while living it up. Aboard the Disney Cruise Line (www. disney.com), for example, extensive salad and vegetarian selections are included on all buffets and quick-service outlets; lighter options, vegetarian dishes, and sugar-free desserts are available at dinner; and the chefs can create specific meals on request. The world-class restaurants of the Norwegian Cruise Line (www.ncl.com) teamed up with *Cooking Light* magazine to bring passengers a selection of dishes high in flavor but low in cholesterol, salt, and fat. And each of Carnival's Fun Ships (www.carnival. com) offers Spa Fare like broiled or roasted poultry and meats, salads with low-fat or fat-free dressings, vegetarian dishes, and desserts prepared with sugar substitutes.

There's even more healthful deliciousness to be found on the high seas:

- In addition to their famed Greenhouse Spa cuisine, an alternative In Balance Menu of light and healthy spa cuisine and healthful shakes (with calories and fat listed) is available throughout the day on all ships in the Holland America Line's five-star fleet (www.hollandamerica.com).

- The *Salute e Benessere*—"Health and Well-being"—Menu on Costa Cruises (www.costacruises.com or 800-33-COSTA) features low-fat, low-carbohydrate, low-calorie, and low-cholesterol courses daily for lunch and dinner (with nutritional information listed), and the vegetarian menu offers a range of variations on Costa's Italian-style cuisine.

- Diet-conscious guests of Radisson Seven Seas (www.rssc.com) may dine from the Well-being Menu at L'Etoile Restaurant aboard the *Paul Gauguin*, or from the Well-being and vegetarian menus aboard the *Seven Seas Voyager*.

- Royal Caribbean (www.royalcaribbean.com or 800-327-6700) designed a ShipShape Menu specifically for health-conscious guests who want to eat like they are on vacation but without the guilt.

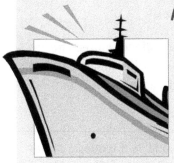

A Floatable Feast

Because cruise-goers are so often bombarded with high-fat "luxury" foods, dieticians with the Physicians Committee for Responsible Medicine (PCRM; www.pcrm.org) investigated the availability of healthful eating options on ten popular cruise lines. The study's results, synopsized below, show that it is possible to eat healthfully on these cruise lines.

PCRM used a four-star scale: one star for serving at least one low-fat, high-fiber entrée for breakfast; one for a vegetarian entrée at lunch and dinner; a bonus star for a vegan (nondairy vegetarian) entrée at lunch and dinner; and one for offering fruit for dessert and snacks.

Carnival Cruise Lines★ ★ ★ ★

Delicious fat-free and cholesterol-free fare such as hot oatmeal and whole-wheat toast with preserves, Jamaican red bean soup with oven-fresh foccacia, a mixed garden and field greens salad, and grilled brochettes of fresh garden vegetables. Website: www.carnival.com.

Norwegian Cruise Line★ ★ ★ ★

Delectable vegetarian selections including Thai pasta salad, zesty Caribbean tofu stir-fry, and daily Indian lunch buffet with entrées like curried vegetables over rice. Website: www.ncl.com.

Royal Caribbean International★ ★ ★ ★

Tasty menu offerings including Tangine vegetable stew, risotto primavera, a California wrap with layers of hummus and roasted vegetables, and low-fat mango strudel. Website www.royalcaribbean.com, or call toll-free 800-327-6700.

Windstar Cruises★ ★ ★ ★

Fresh, light, healthy cuisine, with one or two vegetarian entrée choices at each meal and a range of fresh fruits and vegetables offered for all meals and snacks. Website www.windstarcruises.com, or call 206-281-3535.

Holland America Line★★★

Fresh fruit for dessert and snacks, but lunch and dinner entrée choices routinely high in saturated fat and cholesterol—ask for cholesterol-free vegan meals before embarking. Website: www.hollandamerica.com.

Princess Cruises★★★

Nondairy, cholesterol-free vegetarian entrées available if requested prior to cruise date—but stay away from the misnamed Healthy Choice Menu. Website: www.princesscruises.com.

Celebrity Cruises★★★

Low-fat vegetarian appetizers such as Korean vegetable pancakes or roasted yellow peppers with capers, parsley, and balsamic vinegar, main courses such as vegetable and mushroom pie topped with a cornbread crust, Thai noodle salad with vegetables, or tofu with hummus, tabouli, and tomato. Website: www.celebrity.com.

Crystal Cruises★★★

Vegetarian selections such as potato herb mushroom roll on sautéed leaf spinach, sweet and sour vegetables, grilled asparagus and parsnips, and pressed tomato and basil terrine on a nicoise salad—vegan meals available by pre-cruise request. Website: www.crystalcruises.com.

Disney Cruise Line★★

Vegetarian accommodations provided by headwaiter at dining service hall if requested in advance (recommended to call at least two weeks prior to departure date)—luckily, pasta of the day is often vegetarian or vegan. Website: www.disney.com.

Delta Queen Steamboat Company★★

Vegetarian entrées not guaranteed at lunch and dinner, but vegetarian side orders offered—call ahead with specific requests for healthful choices. Website: www.deltaqueen.com.

FOOD SAFETY

Eating right while traveling isn't just about sticking to a weight-management plan. Eating away from home can also pose a challenge if you suffer from a medical condition such as diabetes, irritable bowel syndrome, or food allergies. And depending on your destination, certain foods can actually make you sick, so it's vital to know what you should and shouldn't eat and drink while you're on the road, or on the boat, or in the air. No one wants to feel sluggish or ill on a trip. Planning ahead, educating yourself, and taking proper precautions are the keys to preventing any health problems that could bring your travels to a sudden halt.

Keep Your Cool

When traveling by car or RV and hauling provisions, it's important to keep your perishables well-chilled in a cooler with ice or refreezable ice-packs. Any uncooked food should be kept cold and cooked promptly when you arrive at your destination. Buy meats daily if possible, instead of storing leftovers. Freezing foods and juices will keep them unspoiled longer. No cooler? Stick with nonperishable items such as crackers, peanut butter, and safely canned or jarred goods. If you buy fresh fruits or vegetables on your journey, peel them yourself and wash them with fresh clean water (see page 106 for water-safety information).

"Waiter, There's a Fly in My Soup—and I'm Allergic to Flies."

An allergy to nuts, chocolate, fish, strawberries, or any other fare presents a potential difficulty when traveling, as you can never be *completely* certain that your meal does not contain your allergen. Even if the waiter says, "No, your food doesn't have peanuts in it," the chef may have used the same utensils in preparing someone else's nut-related dish. It's a risky situation, so it's best to be completely prepared.

First, talk to your allergist or physician about your travel plans (see Chapter 1). Any necessary epinephrine self-injection kit or pen should be kept in your carry-on bag, pocketbook, or pocket at all times, along with the accompanying documentation from the doctor, in case your luggage is lost or delayed. In addition, obtain and wear a MedicAlert or similar bracelet. Several companies sell bracelets and pendants engraved with your medical condition, an ID number, and a twenty-four-hour hotline number that medical professionals can call for information on treating you in an emergency. Alternatively, you can have a regular piece of jewelry engraved with the relevant information yourself.

Packing your own snacks for the trip gives you control over what you're eating, which minimizes your risk of an allergic reaction. Tell everyone including travel companions, flight staff, hotel staff, and restaurant servers about your food allergy, and don't be afraid to repeat yourself often. (*Author's note: I am allergic to shellfish, so every time I eat out I make sure that my friends and my children remember, and that the waiter understands, but the concern is always there. —Lisa*)

If you're traveling to a foreign country, be prepared to explain your allergy to people who don't speak your language. One traveler with food allergies described how a friend had made her a set of cards that read, "Do not give me peanuts—I will die" in an array of languages, so that no matter where she goes, she can show the card to the wait-staff in their native language and feel that she has communicated her situation to the best of her ability. (Of course, this strategy doesn't prevent the cooking staff from using utensils that have already touched the allergen in question, but it is a helpful precaution.)

Ugh . . . My Stomach!

It can ruin your entire trip (or worse) to enjoy a meal and then end up sick. Choose your food with caution and be particularly careful with raw food, which is subject to contamination, especially in areas where hygiene and sanitation are inadequate.

A particularly well-known ailment is traveler's diarrhea or TD, also called "Montezuma's revenge" and "Tut's tummy." Traveler's diarrhea is defined as three or more unformed stools in twenty-four hours in a person from an industrialized nation who is traveling in a less-developed country (see Chapter 2 for more information on TD and other food-borne illnesses). According to the Mayo Clinic (www.mayoclinic.com), high-risk destinations for TD include underdeveloped countries in Latin America, Africa, the Middle East, and Asia. Traveling to southern Europe and a few Caribbean islands also poses some risk. Risk of TD is generally low in northern Europe, Canada, Australia, New Zealand, and the United States.

If you travel to any areas that put you at a high risk for contracting TD, the U.S. Centers for Disease Control (CDC; www.cdc.gov) suggest that you:

- Avoid salads, uncooked vegetables, and unpasteurized milk and milk products such as cheese.

- Only eat food that has been cooked and is still hot. Food that has been allowed to stand for several hours at a lower temperature may have been at risk for bacterial growth.

- Only eat fruit that you have peeled personally.

- Do not eat undercooked or raw meat, fish, or shellfish.

- Be wary of food from street vendors.

- Breastfeed infants under six months of age, or provide them with ready-to-drink formula or formula prepared from commercial powder and boiled water.

- Do not bring perishable seafood with you when you return to the United States from high-risk areas.

If you're a seafood lover, be careful about eating certain species. According to the CDC, the most common type of biotoxin in fish is ciguatoxin, which leads to gastroenteritis (inflammation of the stomach and intestines that may cause diarrhea, vomiting, cramps, and possibly fever) followed by neurological problems. Amberjack, grouper, red snapper, sea bass, and a wide range of tropical reef fish contain ciguatoxin. The flesh of the barracuda is the most toxin-laden, and should always be avoided. Scombroid, another common fish poisoning, occurs in tropical and temperate regions worldwide. High levels of histidine may also be found in the flesh of amberjack, bluefish, herring, bluefin and yellowfin tuna, bonito, mackerel, and mahimahi; if the fish is not refrigerated or preserved properly, the histidine can be converted to histamine and cause flushing, headache, nausea, vomiting, diarrhea, and urticaria (hives) in the unsuspecting consumer.

Cholera

Cholera, a particularly serious form of TD (see Chapter 2), is spread through drinking water, or eating food, that is contaminated with the bacterium *Vibrio cholerae.* Your risk of this intestinal infection is higher if you travel to Latin America, Africa, or Asia. Because the bacteria may live in brackish rivers and coastal waters, shellfish eaten raw can be a source of cholera; some people in the United States, for example, have contracted the illness after eating raw or undercooked shellfish from the Gulf of Mexico.

Typhoid Fever

This infectious illness is usually spread by contamination of food, milk, or water supplies with the bacterium *Salmonella typhi,* either directly by sewage or indirectly by flies or faulty personal hygiene. Fever, abdominal pain, malaise, heat exhaustion, and diarrhea or constipation are common symptoms of typhoid. Without antibiotics, about 15 percent of cases can be fatal, but antibiotic treatment has reduced typhoid mortality to less than 1 percent in the United States. Vaccination of travelers to high-risk or endemic areas is recommended. (see Chapter 1 for more information on typhoid).

Water Wisdom

In areas without chlorination or where hygiene and sanitation are generally poor, the water supply may be contaminated, and it might only be safe to drink the following:

- Beverages made with boiling water (such as tea and coffee)
- Canned or bottled carbonated beverages (including carbonated bottled water and soft drinks)
- Beer and wine

Portable filters currently on the market provide various degrees of protection against water-borne microbes. Remember, however, that in areas where water might be contaminated, ice might also be contaminated and should not be used. The CDC recommends these water-safety tips for people traveling in high-risk areas:

- If ice has been in contact with containers used for drinking water, discard the water and clean the container with soap and hot water.
- Water on the outside of the beverage can or bottle might also be contaminated, so dry any wet cans or bottles before they are opened, and wipe off the area of the can or bottle where you will place your mouth.
- Avoid brushing your teeth with tap water.

The most reliable way to make water safe for drinking (or cooking, or tooth-brushing) is to boil it. Bring it to a vigorous boil for one minute and allow it to cool to room temperature—do not add ice to cool the water. At an altitude higher than 6,562 feet, you should boil the water for three minutes; or, use a chemical disinfection method after boiling the water for one minute. If you will be traveling to an area where you may have to use a chemical method of water disinfection, check out the website www.cdc.gov/travel/food-drink-risks.htm for important instructions. Treating water with iodine, for example, does not protect you from *Cryptosporidium* bacteria unless the water is then allowed to sit for fifteen hours before you drink it. Adding a pinch of salt improves the taste of chemically disinfected water.

Traveler to Traveler

It can be hard to eat when you travel internationally. I always bring a plastic bowl and spoon so I can have cereal in my room for breakfast. I pack some cereal in a plastic-zipped bag and bring a packet of non-fat dried milk. I don't like the whole milk most other countries still use exclusively. I make cold water with ice and then mix some of the powder. I use it in the cereal and in my coffee.

I always travel with a bag of dried fruit (I like apricots and apples) and a bag of almonds. I also bring some Oriental rice snacks for a dose of low-fat carbs. It helps with energy and keeps me from eating the junk that might upset my tummy. And I never go anywhere without my jar of peanut butter. It's got healthy fat and lots of protein. It keeps me from getting hungry. I buy bread when I arrive and have it almost once a day, with fruit on the side, as a meal.

—Daylle Deanna Schwartz

I always bring protein powder, meal-replacement bars, and my shaker with me wherever I travel. That way, I always have something to eat and am not stuck eating something overly fattening. I also make it a point to drink more water than usual when I fly. By staying well hydrated, I don't get as hungry . . . it also helps my metabolism to work more efficiently. When you are dehydrated, your body sends a little signal to your brain telling you that you're hungry—you're really not, but your body knows it can find water in food.

—Melyssa St. Michael

How do you avoid the fast-food frenzy of traveling, especially if you travel by car? Even McDonald's has a McVeggie burger now.

—Tina Tessina, Ph.D.

We always travel with a bag of almonds and a package of Fig Newtons. Good snack foods and reasonably healthy. On trips within the United States, it keeps us from getting hunger pains until we land at our destination.

—Elaine Shimberg

Cereal bars are my number-one choice. They're small, flat, individually wrapped, and, for those who choose wisely, nutritionally sound. They're easy to eat while driving. Trail mix, of course, though less gracefully consumed, usually travels well and provides some nourishment (as do plain raisins or dried fruit). Dry granola-type cereal is fine, too, as is air-popped popcorn. Crackers are indispensable, especially if, before setting out, you make mini peanut butter sandwiches of them. (Peanut butter on whole-wheat bread, of course, is even better from a nutritional standpoint.)

—Chelsea Lowe

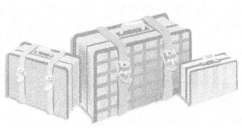

8. S.O.S.: Medical Emergencies

YOU PROBABLY DO NOT WANT TO THINK about the possibility of a medical emergency while you are traveling—nobody does. Read this chapter anyway. It won't be your favorite, but it could be the most important (although we hope you don't ever need to use it).

IS THERE A DOCTOR IN THE HOUSE?

What are the most important things you can do to reduce your chances of having a medical emergency? Use common sense, and prepare. It is easy to overlook such basic guidelines for safe travel as the following:

- Don't drink alcohol excessively on the plane. That can make you very tired and cause you to faint or to be impaired.
- Be aware of your surroundings.
- Don't partake in new activities without guidance from a professional.
- Check your hotel's guidebook for a listing of the "house physician."

How can you prepare for something unforeseen? Well, you really can't, except to be informed and educated before you leave about any possible medical risks that you may encounter *en route* or at your destination. For example, consult your physician(s) and dentist about any preexisting health issues you may have, especially if you haven't had a checkup for quite some time (see Chapter 1). If you have a chronic medical condition or a serious allergy, keep your medication handy, wear a MedicAlert bracelet, and, if you are very concerned or are traveling alone, quietly inform your flight attendant and a fellow traveler about your condition and what to do in an emergency (like a seizure or a hypoglycemia reaction). If you are going to a foreign land that poses a high risk of infection with a disease such as malaria, see a travel physician before you leave, obtain the necessary medication, and take preventive measures against mosquitoes (see Chapter 2).

If you know you will be in need of limited medical attention during your flight, ask your airline if they have qualified companions who could fly with you. (American Airlines, for example, offers the SkycAAre program; see page 9.) Although you'll foot the bill for the companion's seat (at a

A PRIMER FOR TRAVEL EMERGENCIES

Review the following recommendations from the American College of Emergency Physicians (ACEP):

Learn to Recognize Life-threatening Emergencies

Not every cut needs stitches, nor does every burn require advanced medical treatment. If you think someone could suffer significant harm or die unless prompt care is received, that situation is an emergency, and call 9-1-1 or the local hospital for help. (*Author's note: 9-1-1 is only in the United States. Other countries may have different emergency codes or systems, and in undeveloped or third-world countries, you might be essentially on your own. It is best to know ahead of time about the emergency and healthcare facilities at your destination. If you travel with a well-established group or organization like Linblad Expeditions at www.expeditions. com, you are well informed and well protected. —Michael*)

Get help fast when the following warning signs are seen:

- Chest pain lasting two minutes or more (*Author's note: Although this is the ACEP's guideline, I do not feel comfortable putting a time period on chest pain. —Michael*)

- Uncontrolled bleeding

- Sudden or severe pain

- Coughing or vomiting blood

discount) and pay an additional hourly fee for the nurse, it may be cheaper than a full-scale evacuation service.

You may, of course, encounter emergency medical situations that you can't prepare for, such as a heart attack or a broken bone. But you owe it to yourself to analyze your particular conditions and circumstances so that you can do whatever you need to do to stay as healthy as possible when you are traveling. That's what this book is about, after all: to inform you of your risks and help you reduce the chances that you'll become a patient. With this information in hand—carry this book with you—you'll feel confident that you'll know what to do if an emergency arises.

- Difficulty breathing, shortness of breath

- Sudden dizziness, weakness, or change in vision

- Severe or persistent vomiting or diarrhea

- Change in mental status (e.g., confusion, difficulty arousing)

Decide to Act

Be ready, willing, and able to help someone until emergency services arrive. Action can mean anything from calling paramedics, applying direct pressure on a wound, performing CPR, or splinting an injury. Never perform a medical procedure if you're unsure about how to do it.

- Do not move anyone involved in a car accident, serious fall, or is found unconscious unless he or she is in immediate danger of further injury.

- Do not give the victim anything to eat or drink.

- Protect the victim by keeping him or her covered.

- If the victim is bleeding, apply a clean cloth or sterile bandage. If possible, elevate the injury and apply direct pressure on the wound.

- If the victim is not breathing or does not have a pulse, begin rescue breathing or CPR.

—reprinted courtesy of the American College of Emergency Physicians,
Washington, D.C.

In-FLIGHT EMERGENCIES

If you don't think a medical emergency can happen to you while you are in flight, think about this: in 2000, the MedLink Emergency Telemedicine Center in Phoenix, Arizona received over 8,500 calls for in-flight medical emergencies, an all-time high. According to statistics calculated by the center's parent company MedAire, the top categories of medical emergencies among those 8,500 calls were the following:

1. Vasovagal (that is, fainting)   21.4%

2. Gastrointestinal   14.4%

3. Cardiac   12.2%

4. Respiratory   11.0%

5. Neurological   9.7%

What will happen if you are the one in need of emergency medical assistance? There is certainly no guarantee that there will be a doctor onboard. Many years ago, flight attendants were nurses, but unfortunately their training varies today. Most flight attendants know basic cardiopulmonary resuscitation (CPR) and first aid, and also how to use a defibrillator to shock the heart back into normal rhythm during a heart attack. The Federal Aviation Administration (FAA) now requires of all United States airlines that all planes with a flight attendant are to carry a defibrillator; most American carriers operating big planes have been equipped with these devices for years.

United States airlines are also required by the FAA to carry basic medical kits onboard. The medications and other contents of these basic kits are limited, depending on the weight and size of the plane; they include such items as nitroglycerin for heart-related problems, saline solution, intravenous injection equipment, additional drugs, and medications such as Benadryl and epinephrine to counteract allergic reactions. Some airlines, but not all, carry enhanced medical kits that include additional medications and suturing tools.

During an in-flight emergency, the flight staff contacts ground personnel (such as those at MedLink), who assess the severity of the situation and recommend the necessary course of treatment, and it is determined whether or not the plane must be diverted to the nearest airport. Emergencies that do not require a diversion may still require further medical attention; for example, when Joan broke a tooth on an author's tour, the airline called ahead and obtained a dentist's appointment for her that night.

The pain from a toothache or broken tooth can ruin a trip. Dr. James Gutmann, president of the American Association of Endodontics (AAE, www.aae.org), recommends requesting the names of dental professionals and physicians where you are traveling before you leave. "Or, you can contact us on the Internet and we can put you in touch with someone. You don't have to be without access to help."

Here are additional tips from the AAE to help you avoid tooth troubles *en route:*

- Travelers who like to work out on the road should wear a mouth guard to prevent dental injuries.

- If you have a toothache, get it checked before flying. Air pressure changes such as those encountered in plane flight or scuba diving can cause inflammation and worsen the pain.

- While you are away from home, do not bite on hard objects such as the ice in your drink, and be cautious about popcorn kernels and meat bones.

Medical Kits

These specialized medical kits are available from Medex (www.medexassist.com):

- The World Traveler—designed for travelers to developing countries, includes all of the necessities for travel health emergencies as well as supplies for coping with an unsanitary local water supply ($90).

- The Traveler—designed for the frequent traveler, extremely compact and lightweight, includes medication and supplies necessary for any traveler to be prepared in a medical emergency ($42).

- The Dental Medic—designed to help travelers replace lost fillings, loose crowns, and relieve dental pain ($18).

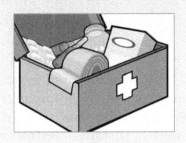

- Do not put aspirin directly on a painful tooth, as that actually burns the tissues. Instead, find a medication based on oil of clove, which will diminish the pain until you can see a dentist or doctor.

Some people find that an over-the-counter medication such as Ambesol is effective for dental pain, but you should only use it until you can see your dentist.

DOMESTIC AND FOREIGN EMERGENCIES

Having access to proper emergency care is vital, especially when you are far from home, and not just on the plane. You may find yourself in a serious situation if you are unfamiliar with your medical insurance policy's requirements or if you take a trip without adequate coverage. If you're traveling on business, check your company's insurance, because different plans have different coverage and most HMOs are restricted. Will they cover an emergency that includes hospitalization and/or evacuation? Most PPOs and HMOs won't.

The American College of Emergency Physicians (ACEP; www.acep.org) suggests asking your insurance provider the following important questions before you travel, whether in the States or internationally:

- How do they provide coverage for a health emergency?

- Do you need permission from your insurance provider to make an emergency department visit?

- Can you go to any emergency department?

- Is your provider available twenty-four hours a day to approve your emergency visit?

- Will your plan pay for emergency department screening exams?

- Once you are admitted, will the physician on duty need authorization from your provider before treating you?

A particularly pressing problem that patients often confront after an emergency visit is the insurance company's refusal to pay for treatment of a condition that turned out not to have been an emergency after all. ACEP president Dr. Larry A. Bedard says, "For example, say you have severe chest pain. Are you having a heart attack? If you sensibly go to an emergency department to find out, before checking with your healthcare insurance provider as some plans require, you may be faced with a big bill after tests determine that you really had indigestion." Some insurance companies may also refuse to pay for emergency services that they have not preauthorized.

Membership in services like MedJet (an air medical evacuation service; www.medjetassistance.com) and Medex (www.medexassist.com; see the inset on page 5) covers expenses such as an evaluation in a medical facility, ground and air transportation, and any physician services or equipment required during an evacuation. You might still need additional travel insurance to cover whatever your existing medical insurance policy doesn't. Travel insurance, which may be purchased per trip or per year, can be used for major medical emergencies and evacuation as well as for baggage or flight delay and for accidental death or dismemberment (however, it is

A Cautionary Tale

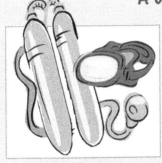

Chris' scuba-diving excursion in the Cayman Islands turned into a life-threatening situation when her body accumulated excess nitrogen and other gases and she got "the bends." This can affect the nervous system, even causing paralysis and death, and she needed medical attention immediately. "An airplane flew me to Grand Cayman Island, which has a decompression chamber, and I slept hooked up to oxygen," says Chris. "I charged the hospital care. The plane, the nurse, and the chamber sent me a bill. I was fortunate that my insurance company paid for everything, except the three days I had to stay to avoid flying."

Chris was fortunate indeed that her insurance company took care of most of her care expenses, and particularly fortunate to have access to and coverage for an evacuation airplane. The cost of international medical transport can be staggering: MedJet Assistance estimates that transports from Europe to the United States average more than $40,000; from the Middle East and South America, $60,000–$85,000; and from the Pacific Rim, $100,000 or more.

Scuba divers should strongly consider membership in Divers Alert Network (DAN; www.diversalertnetwork.org). This organization offers many benefits for divers, including coverage for emergency use of decompression chambers.

important to note that most travel policies do not cover preexisting conditions like high blood pressure or heart ailments that are uncontrolled when you leave for your trip).

Under the Weather Overseas

If you are traveling to foreign soil, don't assume that the country is going to take care of you, or that your medical insurance is necessarily going to travel with you. International financial systems often differ from those in the United States. The ability to pay for medical care when services are rendered is very important, and although most facilities will accept credit cards, you can be "held hostage" until payment is made. Check the overseas provisions of your medical insurance. Find out whether you have to pay up front and then file a claim, and how much is reimbursable.

Another thing to do if you are in need of medical assistance abroad is to contact the local U.S. Embassy or Consulate (record the phone number in your personal health notebook; see Chapter 10). A consular officer can help you find local doctors, dentists, and medical specialists, and the consul will also locate family and friends to inform them of your illness or injury.

Choking

According to the ACEP, nearly 4,000 men, women, and children in the United States die from accidental choking each year. For vital information on assisting victims of choking or drowning, see the following insets about Heimlich maneuvers.

Take the following precautions to prevent choking incidents in young children and infants:

● Supervise mealtimes for young children.

● Do not feed young children hotdogs, nuts, chunks of meat, grapes, hard candy, peanuts, popcorn, chunks of peanut butter, or uncooked vegetables.

● Avoid toys with small parts, and keep other small household items out of reach of young children. Balloons are particularly dangerous.

As for adults, avoid heavy alcohol consumption when eating, and avoid talking and laughing with food in your mouth.

The Heimlich Maneuver
for Choking

A choking victim can't speak or breathe and needs your help immediately. Follow these steps to help a choking victim:

1. From behind, wrap your arms around the victim's waist.

2. Make a fist and place the thumb side of your fist against the victim's upper abdomen, below the ribcage and above the navel.

3. Grasp your fist with your other hand and press into their upper abdomen with a quick upward thrust. Do not squeeze the ribcage; confine the force of the thrust to your hands.

4. Repeat until object is expelled.

Unconscious Victim, or When Rescuer
Can't Reach around Victim

1. Place the victim on back.

2. Facing the victim, kneel astride the victim's hips.

3. With one of your hands on top of the other, place the heel of your bottom hand on the upper abdomen below the ribcage and above the navel.

4. Use your body weight to press into the victim's upper abdomen with a quick upward thrust. Repeat until object is expelled.

5. If the victim has not recovered, proceed with CPR. The victim should see a physician immediately after rescue. Don't slap the victim's back. (This could make matters worse.)

Follow These Steps to Help a Choking Infant

1. Lay the child down, face up, on a firm surface, and kneel or stand at the victim's feet; or hold infant on your lap facing away from you.

2. Place the middle and index fingers of both your hands below his/her ribcage and above the navel.

3. Press into the victim's upper abdomen with a quick upward thrust; do not squeeze the ribcage. Be very gentle. Repeat until object is expelled.

—*reprinted courtesy of the Heimlich Institute, www.heimlichinstitute.org*

The Heimlich Maneuver for Drowning

"You can't get air into the lungs until you get the water out!"

Victim Lying on Ground

1. Place victim on back. Turn face to one side to allow water to drain from mouth.

2. Facing victim, kneel astride victim's hips.

3. With one of your hands on top of the other, place the heel of your bottom hand on the upper abdomen below the ribcage and above the navel.

4. Use your body weight to press into the victim's upper abdomen with a quick upward thrust. Repeat until water no longer flows from the mouth.

—reprinted courtesy of the Heimlich Institute, www.heimlichinstitute.org

Cardiopulmonary Resuscitation

CPR should be started on anyone who is not breathing or who is without a pulse; CPR can keep that person alive until medical help arrives. CPR is a combination of mouth-to-mouth respirations (breaths) and chest compressions that helps oxygenated blood circulate to the brain, heart, and other vital organs. It is also important to note that many public areas in the United States have automatic external defibrillators or AEDs that anyone can use.

To find out how you can learn CPR, visit the websites of the American Heart Association (www.americanheart.org) and the American Red Cross (www.redcross.org) or contact your local chapters of these organizations.

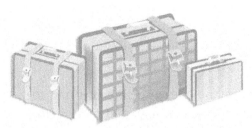

9. Safety Check

WHETHER YOU ARE TRAVELING BY PLANE OR AUTOMOBILE, alone or with a companion, or if your children are traveling solo, the most important safety advice for anyone at any age is to use common sense: don't put yourself into situations where you increase your risk of getting lost, injured, attacked, or killed. If something doesn't feel right, it probably isn't.

Although many safety tips may seem quite obvious, travelers—especially those on vacation—may be looking for a good time while overlooking potential hazards. It's more fun to be laid back than it is to be vigilant, but at an unfamiliar destination or in a foreign land, awareness of your surroundings is a necessity.

Know where you are headed, and know how to get back. Be prepared for a road emergency. Teach your children what to do if you are separated. Be careful with your credit cards and other identification—identity theft occurs worldwide, so don't think it can't happen to you (see page 128). By following the guidelines in this chapter, you'll substantially decrease your chances of jeopardizing your safety and well-being, or that of your family.

Be a Law-Abiding Traveler

Know and obey the laws of the country in which you are traveling. Don't assume that what is acceptable in the United States is acceptable abroad! Get international law information at www.travisa.com.

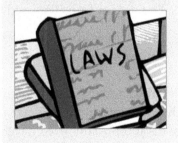

PACKING, PAPERS, AND PROTECTION

Safety while traveling actually begins at home, even before you start to pack. Give careful thought to the documents, clothing, and other items you should bring—and those you should leave behind. (A list of items that are prohibited at airports and on airplanes can be found at www.tsa.gov/public/interapp/editorial/editorial_1012.xml.) If you're traveling internationally, check with the tourism department at your destination to find out what is not allowed into that country.

- Pack wisely. Being overburdened with luggage makes you more of a potential target to thieves.

- Pack clothes that suit the cultural environment. Try not to look touristy or wealthy.

- Don't bring any unnecessary jewelry. Stick to costume jewelry instead. As Sam Fribush of Berman's Jewelers in Ellicott City, Maryland suggests, "This is a good time to bring your jewelry to your jeweler for cleaning and safekeeping."

- Never put personal information on luggage tags (for example, use your business phone number instead of your home phone number).

- Make sure that you have all necessary official documents including your passport, immunization records, letters of information regarding prescriptions and medical equipment, and international driver's license if you'll be driving.

- Protect your passport by carrying it on you at all times. If it's lost or stolen abroad, report the situation immediately to the nearest U.S. Embassy or Consulate and the local police authorities.

- Bring copies of your passport identification page and/or birth certificate with you, as well as extra passport photos.

Your home is also a potential target to thieves while you are away, but there are several things you can do to protect it. First, don't advertise your plans too broadly (you never know who may be listening). Then, when you leave, take the following steps to make sure your home looks lived in, not empty:

- Stop your mail and any regular deliveries.

- Hide empty garbage cans.

- Leave shades and blinds down.

- If possible, put an automatic timer on several lights and a radio.

- Have your property maintained by a trustworthy neighbor or landscaper.

DRIVING AND RIDING SAFETY

No doubt you know to have your vehicle fully inspected (brakes, fluid levels, tires, oil, and so forth) and to check the gas in the tank and the air in the tires (including the spare) before you go. Drivers and passengers alike, however, should take the following extra precautions whenever travel calls for a road trip:

- Bring maps, but leave the touristy stuff in the glove compartment or hidden under something.

- Plan your route before you leave, so you know where you're going and how you're going to get there. If possible, know where the nearest gas station or service station is on your route.

- If you are traveling alone, let someone else know your itinerary.

- Avoid dimly lit streets and alleyways, and avoid traveling during the night if you can, especially in a foreign country.

- Keep your cell phone charged and on you at all times. Don't use your phone while you are driving. If you need to use the phone in an emergency, try to find a safe place to pull off the road; if that isn't possible, use the phone in hands-free or speakerphone mode.

- Whenever you stop overnight, remove bags and other valuables from the car and take them inside your room.

- Never leave your vehicle with the engine running, and lock your doors when you stop.

- Do not leave valuables in your car.

- Never pick up hitchhikers.

- Park in well-lit areas. If you are staying at a hotel where the area is not well lit, use valet parking instead (and make certain that the person parking the car is a legitimate valet).

- *Never—under any circumstances*—leave young children or pets in the car alone.

Whether you are driving your own vehicle or are renting one, it should be equipped with the following tools and first-aid items:

- Basic toolkit
- Blanket(s)
- Complete tire-changing kit: a lug wrench that fits, a jack, spray lubricant to loosen tough lugs, and chocks to hold the car in place when you jack it up to change the tire
- Empty gas can
- Fire extinguisher rated for all types of fires
- First-aid kit (see Chapter 10, and also see the inset Medical Kits on page 113)
- Flashlight and fresh batteries
- Ice scraper and brush
- Jumper cables
- Rain gear (if it's winter, include boots, hat, coat, and gloves)
- Reflective triangles
- Road flares
- Tire sealant
- Traction material such as sand or kitty litter
- Water and nonperishable snacks

If your car breaks down on the highway, pull over to the right side of the road if possible, to get your car out of the flow of traffic and minimize the risk of causing an accident (but see On the Road Abroad, following). Put on your emergency flashers and keep your hood lifted. Have a sign that passersby can read that says "Emergency" or "Send help." Depending on road and weather conditions, stay with your car; but if oncoming cars may hit you, get out and wait in a safer area. Call emergency personnel and let them know where you and your vehicle are located.

On the Road Abroad

Motor-vehicle crashes pose the greatest risk of injury to international travelers, according to the CDC, and the risk of death from motor-vehicle crashes is many times higher outside of the United States. Inadequate roadway design, hazardous conditions, lack of appropriate vehicles and vehicle maintenance, unskilled or inexperienced drivers, inattention to pedestrians and cyclists, and impairment due to alcohol and drugs all contribute to the increased risk of involvement in a vehicle-related crash while visiting other countries.

Consider these important safety tips when driving or riding abroad (some are relevant for domestic drives as well):

- Check with your insurance company before you leave to verify that you're covered for driving while abroad.

- Have a sign prepared that says "Emergency" or "Send help" in the native language, and keep it in the car.

- Be aware of the correct side of the road for driving and for pulling over in case of an emergency—depending on where you are, the right side may not be the "right" side!

- Request a vehicle with safety belts, and use them.

- Request a vehicle equipped with air bags (where available).

- Inspect the vehicle to make sure that the tires, windshield wipers, brakes, and headlights are in good condition.

- Avoid nonessential night driving.

- Avoid drinking alcohol and riding with persons under the influence of alcohol.

- As a passenger, sit in the back seat whenever possible, to minimize the risk of death if an accident should occur.

- Bring a car-safety seat when traveling with a young child.

SAFE HAVEN

When a hotel, motel, or a bed-and-breakfast is going to be your home away from home, you want to be comfortable there, and you also want to be safe. Here are some guidelines for checking out your lodgings and making sure they are secure:

- Start by choosing a reputable establishment through recommendations from your travel agent, friends, auto club, and the like.

- When possible, choose an establishment that uses electronic locks (the combination is changed after each guest leaves).

- When you make your reservation, ask for a room on the lower floors, but not on the first floor (it is easier to break in from a first-floor patio).

- If you are a woman traveling alone or with young children, consider booking the room as "Mr. and Mrs." or with just a first initial and last name.

- Pack a flashlight to keep by your bed along with your room keys, car keys, and wallet or purse.

- Keep an eye on your luggage and wallet when checking in. Don't leave your credit card lying on the check-in counter while you complete your registration.

- Examine the room and make sure that it's been taken care of, nothing has been tampered with, and all window and door locks work properly.

Bikers Be Wary

These are important safety tips for bicycling or motorcycling while on vacation:

- Make sure you observe the rules of the road.

- Wear a safety helmet, and always put a helmet on a young passenger.

- Do not carry infants less than six months old on a bicycle, as they are unable to sit up and their heads may be too wobbly, especially with a helmet.

- Ride only on bike paths or safe streets, not in busy traffic.

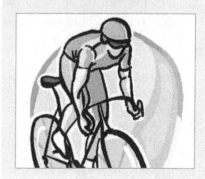

- Make certain that you and your children know where the closest exits are. Check out the exits to make sure the doors are not locked and are easily accessible.

- When you are in your room, secure the door and windows and keep them locked. When you leave your room, do not leave indicators showing that you are out; rather, leave the television or radio on, giving the impression that the room is occupied.

- Stick to well-lit interior hallways, parking lots, and grounds.

- Good security requires that the switchboard not give out room numbers, and the best establishments adhere strictly to this policy.

- If you need to bring anything valuable, store it in the hotel's security vault, and be sure to obtain a receipt for its storage from the staff.

- Local laws in many countries require you to leave your passport at the hotel reception desk overnight so local police officials can check it. If this is the normal procedure at your destination, be sure to obtain a receipt for your passport from the staff.

- If you don't feel comfortable, don't stay.

TRAVELING CHILDREN

Children come with their own set of travel safety challenges. The most important piece of advice is to prepare ahead of time for any possible

Where Am I?

"Immediately upon check-in, get two business cards or matchbooks with the hotel name and address on them. Place one by the phone in the room so you know where you are, and keep the other on you when you leave so you know where to come back to; if you get lost, you'll have the address and phone number handy. There is nothing more frustrating than telling a cab driver to take you to 'the Marriott' and they ask, 'Which one?' That could be one very expensive cab ride. Or if you are in a country where you don't speak the language, you can simply show a taxi driver the matchbook, and you're on your way back to the hotel."

—www.corporatetravelsafety.com

emergencies; that is, make sure you have any necessary prescription or over-the-counter medicine and a first-aid kit handy at all times, and keep the name and number of your pediatrician available in case any questions or concerns arise.

Then, think about your children's behavior at home. Are they curious? Do they have a hard time staying by your side? Your lodging might seem like a safe haven on your travels, but uncovered electrical outlets, improper window locks, and caches of coins or other small items can be danger zones to a baby or young child. Pack some basic childproofing equipment such as plastic socket-plugs, and conduct a complete review of the room to avoid any potential dangers on your vacation—be sure to get down on your children's level and see what they see.

Here are additional child-safety recommendations:

- Check all areas of the room for small choking hazards including coins and paperclips that might have been left behind by previous guests.

- Watch for dangling cords on lamps and for pull-cords on blinds and drapes. Put these cords up higher so your children can't reach them.

- Check the temperature of the running hot water in the sink and bathtub to make sure it doesn't become hot enough to scald your child.

- Place any prescribed or over-the-counter medications out of reach.

- Identify the closest fire exits to your room and show them to your children—don't wait until an emergency to know your escape route.

- Instruct kids not to open hotel room doors to people they don't know.

- Know how to work the room telephone, and bring your cell phone into your room just in case.

If your child needs a crib, bring your own if possible. A few years ago, the Consumer Product Safety Commission (CPSC; www.cpsc.gov) found that 80 percent of cribs examined in ninety hotels and motels in twenty states had at least one safety hazard including soft bedding, loose hardware, and/or adult-sized sheets. According to the CPSC, each year about forty babies suffocate or strangle when they become trapped between broken crib parts or in cribs with older, unsafe designs. Additionally, as many as 3,000 infants die each year from sudden infant death syndrome (SIDS), up to a third of whom may have suffocated on soft bedding such as quilts, comforters, or pillows. The CPSC recommends that a baby less than twelve months old be put to sleep in a crib on his/her back, with no soft bedding. Adult sheets should never be used in a crib because the extra material poses a risk of strangulation and/or suffocation. Hotels and motels should provide crib-sheets in good condition that fit the mattress securely.

Separation Anxiety

The last thing any parents want to think about is something terrible happening to their children. You need to prepare as follows, however, for the possibility that you and your child might be separated during travel:

- Always keep a recent photo of your child in your wallet, and place a photo of yourself in your child's pocket.

- With your older children, review what they should do if they are separated from you. Make sure they know the name and address of the hotel where you are staying. If your last name is different from theirs, make sure they know your name and its spelling as well as their own.

- Make sure your children know about strangers and whom they can trust.

- Do not put your child's name on his/her clothing. Strangers can use this information to lure a child away.

Children and Transportation

Luckily for parents, most kids love airplanes, trains, boats, and buses. To keep them safe in transit, start with the correct child-restraint system. For flight safety, the FAA strongly recommends that children who weigh less than 40 pounds be put into a child-restraint seat appropriate for their weight. Children under the age of two may be carried on the lap of an adult, but a child-safety seat is preferred.

Speaking of restraint, it's very important to keep your little one with you at all times, and under control, in the airport and on the plane (to prevent accidents, do not allow him/her to run through the terminals or down the aisles, especially when food or beverages are being served). When your child needs to take a walk, you need to go along. If your child has any type of medical condition (such as diabetes or a food allergy), notify the flight attendants so they can be aware of any possible complications. And if emergency oxygen masks are deployed, put your mask on first and then put a mask on your child.

Take the following precautions for an older child traveling alone:

- Pack all needed medications in his/her carry-on bag. Inform the flight attendant, if possible, about your child's condition.

- Make sure your child has a list of emergency contact numbers as well as the names, addresses, and phone numbers for you and for the party meeting him/her.

- If you can, escort your child onto the aircraft.

- If your child is old enough, give him/her a cell phone to use for any trip emergencies.

- Make certain that the person meeting your child will have proper identification and will be at the agreed-upon location on time.

IDENTITY THEFT

It is estimated that this year, more than ten million Americans will lose an average of $5,000, but not on a racetrack gamble or the stock market's swinging pendulum: you could be one of those ten million people simply if someone obtains your personal information and uses it to steal your money or your credit. Such a thief might even use your identity to commit another crime and escape prosecution. You may not even know that any of this is happening until it's too late—and it can happen while you're on vacation.

According to the Federal Trade Commission (FTC), 27.3 million Americans have been victims of identity theft in the last five years, including 9.9 million people in 2003 alone. One in four Americans will have his/her identity misused or stolen within the next year. "These numbers are the real thing," says Howard Beales, Director of the FTC's Bureau of Consumer Protection. "For several years, we have been seeing anecdotal evidence that identity theft is a significant problem that is on the rise; now we know. It is affecting millions of consumers and costing billions of dollars. This information can serve to galvanize federal, state, and local law enforcers, the business community, and consumers to work together to combat this menace."

Anyone who uses an ATM or who makes purchases or enters contests on the Internet is a potential victim of identity theft. Common methods of obtaining confidential and/or personal information include hacking into computer systems or posing as someone who is responsible for handling or recording this information. However, according to Jordana Beebe, communications director of Privacy Rights Clearinghouse in San Diego (www.privacyrights.org), "It is very difficult to always find out how the thief gained access because in many cases, law enforcement is too under-staffed to go after the crime."

Prevention, again, is the key to fighting identity theft. Although there is no surefire way to prevent becoming a victim, you can minimize the risks by being very aware of all of your finances and taking certain precau-tions before traveling, as follows:

- Review all of your current financial statements before you leave.

- Know what your outstanding debts are and make a note of the date of this information.

- If possible, obtain and review your credit report (a detailed listing of all of your outstanding debts such as student loans, car loans, mortgage payments, credit card debt, and so on) before you leave and again after you return home. These reports are updated monthly, and you should check yours regularly if possible. You can do this at www.equifax.com.

- Notify your credit card company of your travel plans so that they can make a notation on your account and be suspicious of any odd activity (for example, if you tell them that you are traveling to France and then they notice that several purchases are being made with your card in Texas, this may be an important indicator of trouble).

Inviting Trouble

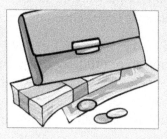

"Traveling with extra checks in your wal-let, credit cards you don't need, or a list of all your bank account numbers is almost an invitation for identity theft," says Frank Abagnale, Jr. (the subject of the movie *Catch Me If You Can*). "Too often, identity thieves start their work with a stolen wal-let or purse. The more information in your wallet or purse, the easier it is for them to steal your identity."

—*PR Newswire*, Norwalk, CT, Dec. 11, 2004

- If a house sitter, pet sitter, or anyone else will be in your home while you're away, lock up any documents that are imprinted with your Social Security, credit card, or other identifying numbers.

Follow these additional suggestions to prevent identity theft during your travels:

- At airports, check out the photo ID of anyone who requests your ID, and don't show your ID to someone who you suspect might not be a legitimate airport or airline employee.

- Never carry a list of your bank account numbers in your wallet or purse.

- Never carry your Social Security card or number on a trip.

- "Don't put your Social Security Number or driver's license number on your checks." —Identity Theft Resource Center, www.idtheftcenter.org

- Store any copies of documents that you brought with you that may have personal information on them in the hotel safe, along with any other valuables. Do not leave these documents exposed in your room.

- A common scam is for thieves to call hotel rooms, claim to be the front desk staff, and ask for verification of a credit card number. Never give out any credit card information on an incoming call; instead, tell the caller that you will bring the number to the desk in person (and don't ask for a number to call back, because a thief can easily make one up). If you find out the call was a scam, report it to the hotel's management and to the police.

- If you use your credit cards, keep all of your receipts (in your suitcase or carry-on bag, *not* in your purse or wallet) to take home and compare to your next statement(s).

- Call the customer service number for your account(s) regularly, and compare balances (when using a phone to check a balance, hide the keypad so nobody can read the numbers over your shoulder). If something doesn't seem right, call a representative at the credit card company immediately.

Finally, when you get home from your trip and are throwing out your receipts and other papers, use a crosscut shredder to assure that anything with your account numbers and other personal information on it is properly destroyed and cannot be pieced together (or, if you have a fireplace, burn the paperwork instead). It is also very important to pay close attention to all financial statements you receive after you get home. If you see any transaction that you do not believe you made, contact the creditor or other institution company immediately. According to the FTC survey mentioned above, some consumers weren't aware of the fraud on their accounts until six months after the fraud occurred. How can this happen? Easily: many consumers who charge items on credit fail to really examine the bill, and consequently don't notice anything until their credit card company calls or a discrepancy appears on their credit report.

If you're particularly concerned about having your identity stolen, you can purchase identity-theft insurance through most insurance carriers or credit bureaus. This insurance provides privacy and fraud protection and helps you to monitor and manage your credit information. Consider obtaining a policy in advance of your trip. If someone steals your identity

Insuring Your Identity

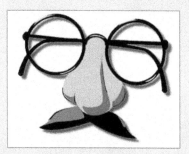

Identity-theft insurance is designed to help you recover both your identity and your recovery-related expenses, from taking time off work and paying a lawyer for civil suits to notary and other fees and refiling for loans. According to the Insurance Information Institute (III; www.iii.org), these policies cost between $25 and $50 on average (with annual premiums or monthly fees, depending on your package selection), provide $15,000–$25,000 worth of coverage, and are offered by the following companies:

- American International Group, www.aig.com
- Chubb Group of Insurance Companies, www.chubb.com
- Encompass Insurance, www.encompassinsurance.com
- Farmers Group, Inc., www.farmers.com
- Travelers Insurance, www.travelers.com

while you are traveling and damages result, the insurance will cover some of your expenses in reestablishing your identity, including legal fees and lost wages (see the inset Insuring Your Identity on page 131).

If you think you've become a victim of identity theft, act immediately as follows:

1. Close the accounts that you believe have been victimized.

2. Contact the fraud departments of any one of the three major credit bureaus to place a fraud alert on your credit file: Equifax, www.equifax.com or 800-685-1111; Experian, www.experian.com or 888-397-3742; or TransUnion, www.transunion.com (no phone number available). According to the FTC, "The fraud alert requests creditors to contact you before opening any new accounts or making any changes to your existing accounts. As soon as the credit bureau confirms your fraud alert, the other two credit bureaus will be automatically notified to place fraud alerts, and all three credit reports will be sent to you free of charge."

3. Once you have completed those steps, file a police report and file a report with the FTC (www.ftc.gov; the FTC's database of identity theft cases is used by law-enforcement agencies for investigations).

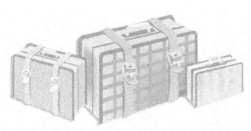

10. Your Personal Health Notebook

THIS CHAPTER PROVIDES A COMPREHENSIVE TRAVEL "TO-DO LIST" and a convenient place for you to record all of the important information we've discussed in the previous chapters. The checklists include reminders to photocopy some of that information to give to your emergency contacts as well. *Note:* If you are traveling with a companion, spouse, and/or children, fill out the relevant portions for *each* traveler.

Using this chapter will ensure that your medical and other travel-related information is well organized and complete, and packing this book in your carry-on bag (or keeping it with you at all times) will ensure that your "personal health notebook" and other useful information is always handy in case of any question or emergency on your trip. Happy—and healthy—trails to you!

🚃 ✈ 🚐 MY TRAVEL LOG 🚗 ⛴ 🚚

Traveler _____

Date(s) of Trip _____

Mode(s) of Travel _____

_____

Destination(s) _____

_____

_____

Type(s) of Lodging _____

_____

_____

_____

Type(s) of Activities _____

_____

_____

_____

_____

_____

_____

_____

MY TRAVEL LOG

Traveler _____

Date(s) of Trip _____

Mode(s) of Travel _____

_____

Destination(s) _____

_____

_____

Type(s) of Lodging _____

_____

_____

_____

Type(s) of Activities _____

_____

_____

_____

_____

_____

_____

_____

MY TRAVEL LOG

Traveler _____

Date(s) of Trip _____

Mode(s) of Travel _____

_____

Destination(s) _____

_____

_____

Type(s) of Lodging _____

_____

_____

_____

Type(s) of Activities _____

_____

_____

_____

_____

_____

_____

_____

MY TRAVEL LOG

Traveler _____

Date(s) of Trip _____

Mode(s) of Travel _____

_____

Destination(s) _____

_____

_____

Type(s) of Lodging _____

_____

_____

_____

Type(s) of Activities _____

_____

_____

_____

_____

_____

_____

_____

CONTACT NAMES AND NUMBERS

❑ *Record the contact information indicated below for reaching family, friends, neighbors, house sitters, pet sitters, doctors, and the like.*

In case of emergency, contact the following people:

_____ Phone _____

_____ Phone _____

_____ Phone _____

_____ Phone _____

_____ Phone _____

Other emergency contact information:

Physician _____ Phone _____

Pediatrician _____ Phone _____

Travel physician _____ Phone _____

Obstetrician_____ Phone _____

Dentist_____ Phone _____

Ophthalmologist _____ Phone _____

Optometrist_____ Phone _____

Veterinarian_____ Phone _____

Other _____ Phone _____

Other _____ Phone _____

Other _____ Phone _____

Other _____ Phone _____

❏ *International travelers: check the relevant consular information sheet(s) at the U.S. Department of State's website (www.state.gov) for the address and phone number of the U.S. embassy and consulate at your destination(s), and record below.*

Address _____   Phone _____

Address _____   Phone _____

Address _____   Phone _____

❏ *Photocopy the trip summary and the contact lists above; give one copy to your emergency contact(s) and keep a copy for your carry-on bag, pocketbook, or pocket.*

MEDICAL PROFILE

❏ *Record the following information about any existing health conditions (include allergies) and any current nonprescription or prescription medications (include the brand name and the generic name), confirming details with your physician(s) as necessary (see Appointments section).*

Condition _____   Medication _____
                                    Physician/
Dosage _____   Phone _____

Condition _____   Medication _____
                                    Physician/
Dosage _____   Phone _____

Condition _____   Medication _____
                                    Physician/
Dosage _____   Phone _____

Condition _____   Medication _____
                                    Physician/
Dosage _____   Phone _____

Any changes in effectiveness at high altitudes?   ☐ YES   ☐ NO

If YES, describe: _____

Any adverse interactions with sunlight?   ☐ YES   ☐ NO

If YES, describe: _____

Medical
Equipment _____

_____

Blood Type _____

❏ *Fill in the following chart, consulting your physician(s) as necessary.*

IMMUNIZATION STATUS

❏ *Check any of the following childhood vaccinations that you have received:*

☐ Measles   ☐ Mumps   ☐ Rubella
☐ Varicella   ☐ Hepatitis B series   ☐ Polio series
☐ Other(s) _____

❏ *Fill in the latest dates that you received the following immunizations:*

Tetanus/Diphtheria _____

Hepatitis A #1 _____   # 2 _____

Hepatitis B #1 _____   #2 _____   #3 _____

Twinrix A/B #1 _____   #2 _____   #3 _____

Adult Polio booster _____

Typhoid Fever _____   ( ) pills   ( ) shot

Meningococcal Meningitis _____

Japanese Encephalitis series _____

Yellow Fever _____ (*Note:* carry Yellow Card with your passport)

Influenza _____

Pneumonia _____

Rabies series _____ (*Note:* need two more shots if exposed to rabies)

❏ *Show your filled-in Immunization Status chart to the healthcare provider at the Travel Clinic (see Appointments, below).*

❏ *Photocopy your medical information; give one copy to your emergency contact(s) and keep a copy for your carry-on bag or pocketbook.*

❏ *Visit www.personalmd.com if you wish to set up an online health database and/or use the RemindRx service for any scheduling or other reminders.*

APPOINTMENTS

❏ *Make appointments with physicians and specialists (and obtain any additional medical advice) at least six weeks prior to your departure (if possible), and record all of the information indicated below.*

❏ *Diabetic travelers or others using syringes or lancets: see Chapter 1 for medication and documentation details, and obtain any necessary paperwork from your doctor.*

❏ *Disabled travelers: see Chapter 1 for equipment and documentation details, and obtain any necessary paperwork from your doctor.*

PRIMARY CARE PHYSICIAN

Name _____ Phone _____

Appointment date and time_____

❏ *Pre-trip questions:*

1. Immunizations needed/suggested? (see Immunization Status chart in Medical Profile, above)

2. Insect sting emergency allergy kit prescription needed?

3. _____

4. _____

5. _____

❏ *Obtain any needed prescription(s), along with a document from the prescrib - ing physician listing the physician's name, address, and phone number, the medication's brand name and generic name, and the reason(s) for its use.*

❏ *Schedule post-trip checkup.*

Appointment date and time_____

❏ *Post-trip questions:*

1. _____

2. _____

3. _____

4. _____

TRAVEL PHYSICIAN/CLINIC

Name _____ Phone _____

Appointment date and time _____

❏ *Pre-trip questions:*

1. Immunizations needed/suggested? (see Immunization Status chart in Medical Profile, above)

2. _____

3. _____

4. _____

❏ *Obtain any needed prescription(s), along with a document from the prescribing physician listing the physician's name, address, and phone number, the medication's brand name and generic name, and the reason(s) for its use.*

❏ *Schedule post-trip checkup.*

Appointment date and time _____

❏ *Post-trip questions:*

1. _____

2. _____

3. _____

4. _____

DENTIST

Name _____ Phone _____

Appointment date and time _____

❏ *Pre-trip questions:*

1. _____

2. _____

3. _____

4. _____

OBSTETRICIAN/GYNECOLOGIST

Name _____   Phone _____

Appointment date and time _____

❑ *Pre-trip questions:*

1. If I'm pregnant, am I approved to fly/travel? _____

2. _____

3. _____

4. _____

❑ *If pregnant, make sure to fill in the "Nearest Hospital" information in the Destination(s) section of this chapter.*

❑ *If needed, obtain a letter from the obstetrician giving you permission to fly, along with the obstetrician's name, address, and phone number.*

❑ *Obtain any needed prescription(s), along with a document from the prescribing physician listing the physician's name, address, and phone number, the medication's brand name and generic name, and the reason(s) for its use.*

❑ *Schedule post-trip checkup.*

Appointment date and time _____

❑ *Post-trip questions:*

1. _____

2. _____

3. _____

4. _____

OPHTHALMOLOGIST

Name _____   Phone _____

Appointment date and time _____

❑ *Pre-trip questions:*

1. _____

2. _____

3. _____

4. _____

❏ *Obtain any needed prescription(s), along with a document from the prescribing physician listing the physician's name, address, and phone number, the medication's brand name and generic name, and the reason(s) for its use.*

OPTOMETRIST

Name _____ Phone _____

Appointment date and time _____

❏ *Pre-trip questions:*

1. _____

2. _____

3. _____

4. _____

❏ *Obtain a copy of your existing prescription, or any needed prescription(s), for glasses and/or contact lenses.*

❏ *Obtain any needed glasses (or an extra pair) and/or contact lenses.*

SPECIALIST #1

Name _____ Phone _____

Appointment date and time _____

❏ *Pre-trip questions:*

1. _____

2. _____

3. _____

4. _____

❑ *Obtain any needed prescription(s), along with a document from the prescrib-ing physician listing the physician's name, address, and phone number, the medication's brand name and generic name, and the reason(s) for its use.*

SPECIALIST #2

Name_____   Phone_____

Appointment date and time_____

❑ *Pre-trip questions:*

1. _____

2. _____

3. _____

4. _____

❑ *Obtain any needed prescription(s), along with a document from the prescrib-ing physician listing the physician's name, address, and phone number, the medication's brand name and generic name, and the reason(s) for its use.*

SPECIALIST #3

Name_____   Phone_____

Appointment date and time_____

❑ *Pre-trip questions:*

1. _____

2. _____

3. _____

4. _____

❑ *Obtain any needed prescription(s), along with a document from the prescrib -ing physician listing the physician's name, address, and phone number, the medication's brand name and generic name, and the reason(s) for its use.*

SPECIALIST #4

Name_____   Phone_____

Appointment date and time_____

❏ *Pre-trip questions:*

1. _____

2. _____

3. _____

4. _____

❏ *Obtain any needed prescription(s), along with a document from the prescribing physician listing the physician's name, address, and phone number, the medication's brand name and generic name, and the reason(s) for its use.*

VETERINARIAN

Name_____ Phone_____

Appointment date and time_____

❏ *Pre-trip questions:*

1. Does my pet need any vaccinations?
   ☐ Rabies   ☐ Lyme   ☐ Other _____

   _____

2. If this is international travel, what documents do I need for my pet?

   _____

   _____

3. If this is international travel, are there any quarantine requirements?

   _____

4. _____

5. _____

❏ *If necessary, obtain a written statement from your veterinarian of your pet's health and vaccination status, also listing the vet's name, address, and phone number.*

❏ *Obtain any needed prescription(s), along with a document from the prescribing physician listing the physician's name, address, and phone number, the medication's brand name and generic name, and the reason(s) for its use.*

INSURANCE

❏ *Check your current medical insurance for travel coverage, and record the information indicated below.*

❏ *Questions to ask:*

1. _____

2. _____

3. _____

4. _____

MEDICAL INSURANCE COMPANY #1

Name _____   Phone _____

Policy number _____

Notes_____

MEDICAL INSURANCE COMPANY #2

Name _____   Phone _____

Policy number _____

Notes_____

MEDICAL INSURANCE COMPANY #3

Name _____   Phone _____

Policy number _____

Notes_____

❏ *Purchase traveler's and evacuation insurance if needed, and record the information indicated below.*

❏ *Questions to ask:*

1. _____

2. _____

3. _____

4. _____

TRAVELER'S INSURANCE COMPANY #1

Name _____ Phone _____

Policy number _____

Notes _____

TRAVELER'S INSURANCE COMPANY #2

Name _____ Phone _____

Policy number _____

Notes _____

❑ *Photocopy the above insurance information, your insurance policies, and your insurance ID card(s); give one copy to your emergency contact(s) and keep a copy for your carry-on bag or pocketbook.*

SUPPLY CHECK

❑ *Obtain enough of your prescription medication(s) for your entire trip—and keep prescription medications in their original, labeled containers for travel.*

❑ *International travelers: get your destination country's embassy or consulate contact information from U.S. Department of State's website at www.state.gov, record it below, and contact the embassy or consulate to find out about any paperwork or forms that are needed to bring medication into that country.*

EMBASSY/CONSULATE

Phone _____ Website _____

Notes _____

❑ *International travelers: check the consular information sheet(s) at www.state.gov for information regarding traveling with medication.*

Notes _____

❑ *Diabetic travelers or others using syringes or lancets: see Chapter 1 for medication and documentation details.*

❑ *Disabled travelers: see Chapter 1 for equipment and documentation details.*

❏ *Photocopy your prescription(s), medications list, and the completed paperwork that you need in order to travel with medication; give one copy to your emergency contact(s) and keep a copy for your carry-on bag or pocketbook.*

❏ *International travelers: photocopy your passport identification page and/or birth certificate, and keep your extra passport photos, for your carry-on bag or pocketbook.*

❏ *Review the following supply lists and circle the items you need to obtain for your trip.*

FIRST-AID KIT

(*Note:* Medical kits are also available from Medex; see page 113.)

Absorbent cotton and/or gauze pads

Alcohol swabs

Antiseptic

Bandages (including triangular bandage, sling, and splint)

Band-aids

Blanket

Burn ointment and dressings

Butterfly closures

Cotton swabs

Disinfectant

Disposable gloves

First-aid instruction booklet

Flashlight

Hot/cold packs

Insect sting emergency allergy kit, and copy of prescription

Knife or scissors (only permissible if *not* traveling by air)

Moleskin (for foot blisters or reducing friction under casts or bandages)

Safety pins

Steri-strips

Tape (hypoallergenic and waterproof)

Tweezers

HEALTH SUPPLIES

(*Note:* This list repeats some items listed above in First-Aid Kit.)

Allergy medication

Altitude-sickness medication

Antacid

Antihistamine

Chewing gum (for restoring ear air pressure when flying)

Cold remedy

Collapsible cup

Compression stockings

Contact lenses and solution, and copy of lens prescription

Contraceptives (including condoms)

Cough medicine

Decongestant

Dental floss

Diarrhea medication

Disposable gloves

Disposable moist towelettes

Duct tape (especially useful in the wilderness)

Eardrops (for earache or ear infection)

Earplugs

Eye mask or blindfold

Feminine-hygiene products

Fever reducer

Flip-flops (for the shower)

Ginger (for nausea/motion sickness)

Glasses (and an extra pair) and copy of glasses prescription

Hand sanitizer

Hat

Insecticide such as permethrin (and/or insecticide-impregnated clothing)

Insect repellent such as a DEET-containing product

Insect sting emergency allergy kit, and copy of prescription

Jet lag remedy

Knife or scissors (only permissible if *not* traveling by air)

Lavender oil (for promoting relaxation or sleep)

Laxatives

Light box/light visor/other (for fighting jet lag)

Lip balm

Malaria medication

MedicAlert bracelet

Melatonin (for fighting jet lag)

Menstrual cramp medication

Moleskin (for foot blisters or reducing friction under casts or bandages)

Mosquito netting

Mouthwash

Nausea/motion sickness medication

Oral/rectal thermometer

Pain medication

Pillbox with daily compartments

Plastic bottle for preparing oral rehydration solution

Plastic bottle for preparing purified water

Pressure-point bracelet (for nausea/motion sickness)

Safety pins, rubber bands, related items

Sewing needle, thread, related items

Shampoo

Soap

Sunscreen with SPF of 15 or higher

Syringes/needles/lancets, with letter of authorization

Toothache medication

Topical itching medication such as hydrocortisone cream or calamine lotion

Topical skincare products (antibiotic, antiseptic, and antifungal)

Tweezers

Urinary tract/vaginal infection medication

UV-protective sunglasses

Vaseline or similar gel/ointment

Vitamins

Water purification kit/filters and/or iodine tablets (see page 00 about water treatment)

RESERVATIONS

❏ *Make all needed reservations and record information, including phone numbers, below.*

AIRPLANE RESERVATION(S)

_____

_____

_____

_____

OTHER TRANSPORTATION RESERVATION(S)

_____

_____

_____

RENTAL VEHICLE RESERVATION(S)

_____

_____

_____

LODGING RESERVATION(S)

_____

_____

_____

OTHER RESERVATIONS(S)

_____

_____

_____

❏ *Photocopy your trip itinerary, reservation information, and any ticket information; give one copy to your emergency contact(s) and keep a copy for your carry-on bag or pocketbook.*

AIRPORT(S) AND OTHER TRANSPORT STATIONS

❑ *Research where to eat healthfully, exercise, relax, and have fun while you're in transit, and record the information indicated below.*

TERMINAL #1

Name _____   Website/Phone _____

Notes _____

_____

TERMINAL #2

Name _____   Website/Phone _____

Notes _____

_____

TERMINAL #3

Name _____   Website/Phone _____

Notes _____

_____

TERMINAL #4

Name _____   Website/Phone _____

Notes _____

_____

❑ *Disabled travelers: check www.tsa.gov for up-to-date transportation information.*

Notes _____

_____

_____

_____

_____

DESTINATION(S)

❑ *Research the following destination information and record below.*

HEALTH CLUBS/GYMS/WORKOUT FACILITIES/SPAS
(At Lodging or Nearby)

Gym Membership #1 _____

Membership   Contact
number_____   information_____

Gym Membership #2 _____

Membership   Contact
number_____   information_____

ATM LOCATIONS IN THE AREA

_____

_____

NEAREST HOSPITAL

_____

_____

Area Hospitals Accepting Medical Insurance (if applicable):

_____

_____

❑ *Check the websites of the Centers for Disease Control and Prevention (www.cdc.gov) and the World Health Organization (www.who.int/ith) to read the most up-to-date health advisories for your destination(s).*

Notes_____

_____

❑ *International travelers: check the relevant consular information sheet(s) at the U.S. Department of State's website www.state.gov for the address and phone number of the U.S. embassy and consulate at your destination(s).*

Notes_____

_____

THE HOME FRONT

❏ *Notify your neighbor or house sitter of your travel plans, and record his/her name and phone number here:*

Neighbor _____   Phone _____

❏ *Arrange for a pet sitter or pet boarding, and record the sitter's/boarder's name and phone number here:*

Pet Sitter_____   Phone _____

❏ *Notify your credit card companies of your travel plans, and record your account numbers and customer service phone numbers here:*

Account _____   Phone _____

Account _____   Phone _____

Account _____   Phone _____

❏ *Prepay your upcoming bills or make other payment arrangements.*

❏ *Suspend your mail and newspaper deliveries or arrange for pickup.*

❏ *Notify your home security system company of your travel plans, and record the company's name and phone number here:*

Security
Company_____   Phone _____

❏ *Reschedule any regular appointments such as gardener, housekeeper, and the like (do NOT tell them that you will be away, only that you need to reschedule).*

❏ *International travelers: obtain an international driver's license if needed.*

❏ *Get cash and/or traveler's checks and/or foreign currency.*

❏ *Check your cell phone service for coverage and use at your destination(s).*

❏ *Arrange to have your email checked while you are away and/or check it from your destination(s).*

❏ *Replace/recharge the batteries in your camera, laptop, watch, and such.*

❏ *Confirm your flight information at least seventy-two hours beforehand.*

❏ *Check the weather at your destination(s).*

❏ *Have your car examined (windshield-wiper and other fluids, oil, brakes, and so forth).*

❏ *Fill your car's gas tank the day before you leave.*

❏ *Clean out your wallet (leave any nonessential credit cards and such at home).*

❏ *Check your refrigerator and throw out any items that will expire or spoil while you're gone.*

❏ *Unplug appliances, lamps, computer, and the like and/or set some lights and a radio on a timer to create a "lived-in" illusion while you're away.*

❏ *Leave key and instructions for your neighbor or house sitter.*

❏ *Leave key and instructions for your pet sitter.*

❏ *Set your security system.*

OTHER THINGS TO TAKE CARE OF ON THE HOME FRONT

_____

_____

_____

_____

_____

_____

_____

_____

_____

_____

_____

_____

PACKING

Note: Do *not* pack or bring prohibited items to the airport (review list at www.tsa.gov/public/interapp/editorial/editorial_1012.xml).

❏ *Diabetic travelers or others using syringes or lancets: see Chapter 1 for packing and screening details.*

❏ *Disabled travelers: see Chapter 1 for packing and screening details.*

❏ *Remember your child's car-safety seat (for the airplane as well as the car) and stroller (which can usually be stowed in an airplane's overhead compartment).*

IN CHECKED OR SHIPPED LUGGAGE

Note: Do *not* pack cash, medication, jewelry, laptops, or any valuables in your checked or shipped luggage (keep them in your carry-on bag, pocketbook, or pocket; see below).

Note: Do *not* pack the originals or copies of any important documents in your checked or shipped luggage (keep them in your carry-on bag, pocketbook, or pocket; see below).

Note: Do *not* pack undeveloped film or cameras containing film in your checked luggage, as the screening equipment used will damage undeveloped film (keep them in your carry-on bag, pocketbook, or pocket; see below).

❏ *Pack clothes that suit the cultural environment—try not to look touristy or wealthy*

❏ *Workout clothes and gear*

❏ *Your own bicycle helmet, if you plan to bicycle (for better fit, especially with kids)*

❏ *Pillbox with daily compartments*

❏ *Flashlight*

❏ *Socket-plugs and other basic childproofing equipment*

IN CARRY-ON BAG

❏ *This book*

❏ *Travel itinerary*

❏ *Hotel and other reservation confirmation(s)*

❏ *Rental car/shuttle information*

❏ *Other travel documents*

❏ *Emergency contact phone numbers*

❏ *Insurance documents*

❏ *Medical documents including immunization record (if required)*

❏ *Any necessary letters from physicians*

❏ *Official documents regarding prescriptions and medical equipment*

❏ *Documents from veterinarian*

❏ *Traveler's checks*

❏ *Copies of your passport identification page and/or birth certificate*

❏ *Extra passport photos*

❏ *All necessary medications and health supplies (including such items as knee supports, oral retainer, and contact lens solution)*

❏ *Hand sanitizer*

❏ *Disposable moist towelettes*

❏ *Pressure-point bracelet*

❏ *Snacks and beverages*

❏ *Reading material, music, and other entertainments*

❏ *Laptop computer*

❏ *Camera, film, and batteries*

❏ *Extra batteries (in a plastic bag)*

❏ *Change of clothes*

❏ *Pajamas*

❏ *Workout clothes for exercising en route*

❏ *Hat*

❏ *Breakables or gifts*

IN POCKETBOOK OR POCKET

Note: Keep airline boarding pass(es) and your photo ID handy for all security checkpoints—an ID-holder that hangs around your neck is especially convenient.

❏ *Wallet (see In Wallet, following)*

❏ *Passport (if required)*

❏ *Visas (if required)*

❏ *Yellow Card (keep with your passport)*

❏ *Airline/other transportation tickets*

❏ *Place a photo of yourself in your traveling child's pocket*

❏ *Glasses*

❏ *UV-protective sunglasses*

❏ *Chewing gum*

❏ *Lip balm, Vaseline, similar gel/ointment*

❏ *Cell phone*

❏ *PDA*

❏ *Money clip*

IN WALLET

Note: Never carry a list of your account numbers in your wallet or pocket-book, and never carry your Social Security card or number on a trip.

❏ *Photo ID (alternatively, keep in an ID-holder that hangs around your neck)*

❏ *Medical insurance ID/policy cards*

❏ *ATM debit card*

❏ *Credit card(s)*

❏ *Long-distance calling card*

❏ *Driver's license (and international driver's license if needed)*

❏ *Money including small bills for tipping or vending machines*

❏ *Recent photo of your traveling child/children*

WHAT TO WEAR

Note: Do *not* wear metal-containing apparel (shoes, clothing, or accessories) that may set off the alarm on a metal detector. Prior to entering screening checkpoint(s), place keys, loose change, lighter, and large jewelry/belt buckle/metal hair ornaments in carry-on bag or pocketbook.

❏ *Clothes that suit the cultural environment—try not to look touristy or wealthy*

❏ *Comfortable, appropriate shoes (see Chapter 5)*

❏ *MedicAlert bracelet*

ADDITIONAL NOTES

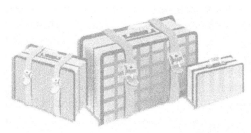

Resources

Some of these resources have been mentioned in this book, others come highly recommended from travelers, and some are just quirky websites about traveling and related topics that you might find helpful or interesting.

WEBSITES

Cruising

www.caribbean-on-line.com/cruise-lines

www.cdc.gov/nceh/vsp/scores/legend.htm – CDC's Green Sheet for Cruises

www.cruisediva.com – CruiseDiva

www.cruise-links.com/CruiseMagazines.htm

www.cruisereviews.com

www.raynorshyn.com/cruises

Health and Fitness Information

www.aaos.org – American Academy of Orthopaedic Surgeons

www.acefitness.org – American Council on Exercise

www.AmericasHealthiestMom.com – "America's Healthiest Mom" Jyl Steinback

www.antijetlagdiet.com/index.asp – Argonne Anti-Jet Lag Diet

www.cdc.gov/travel – Centers for Disease Control and Prevention www.diabetes.org – American Diabetes Organization

www.drweil.com – Dr. Andrew Weil

www.efit.com

www.elainepetrone.com – stress-reduction expert Elaine Petrone

www.fearlessflying.net – Institute of Psychology for Air Travel

www.fitforbusiness.com

www.fitnesszone.com

www.healthclubs.com

www.healthyback.com

www.ihrsa.org or cms.ihrsa.org – International Health, Racquet, and Sportsclub Association

www.istm.org – International Society of Travel Medicine

www.makoa.org

www.medexassist.com – Medex, comprehensive traveler's coverage and assistance

www.medjetassistance.com – MedJet

www.myfitnessexpert.com

www.nia.nih.gov – National Institute on Aging

www.personalmd.com – PersonalMD

www.sleepfoundation.org – National Sleep Foundation

www.usms.org – United States Masters Swimming

www.who.int/ith – World Health Organization

www.ymca.net

Luggage

www.samsonitecompanystores.com – Samsonite

www.travel-goods.org – Travel Goods Association

www.travelonbags.com – Travelon bags (or 800-537-5544)

Reservations, Schedules, and Other Logistics

www.amtrak.com

www.expedia.com – Expedia

www.go-today.com

www.hotels.com

www.hotwire.com – Hotwire

www.orbitz.com – Orbitz

www.seatexpert.com – "the unofficial site for all your airline seat selection needs," advice on the most desirable seats as well as which seats to avoid at all cost

www.seatguru.com – helps airline travelers locate seats with laptop power, Internet access, extra legroom, and in-seat video screens

www.travelocity.com – Travelocity

www.tripadvisor.com

www.webflyer.com

Shipping

www.golfbagshipping.com – Golf Bag Shipping

www.luggageconcierge.com – Luggage Concierge

www.luggagefree.com – Luggage Free

Travel Guides, Tips, and More

www.aaa.com – American Automobile Association

www.brianbrawdy.com – outdoor-travel expert Brian Brawdy

www.camp-a-roo.com – Camp-a-Roo

www.fodors.com – access to Fodor's guidebooks, magazine, and other travel information

www.flyertalk.com – chat with other frequent flyers

www.flying-with-disability.org

www.freetraveltips.com

www.frequentflyer.oag.com – Frequent Flyer by Official Airline Guides (OAG), catering to the frequent business traveler but a great resource for all travelers (*Author's note: My favorite—could it be because I write for them? – Lisa*); the OAG Data division operates the world's most comprehensive flight schedule database (collecting the schedules of over 930 airlines, holding over 1.5 million flight sectors, and verifying, quality-checking, and processing them for distribution throughout the airline and travel industries), and the OAG Publishing division is known worldwide for its Official Airline Guides as well as for providing relevant and reliable information to travelers, travel organizers, government agencies, and the cargo industry

www.hikerwriter.com – a great resource for backpackers, hikers, and adventurers, by Karen Berger (author of several outdoor-adventure books including *Hiking the Triple Crown: How to Hike America's Longest Trails, The Pacific Crest Trail: A Hiker's Companion,* and *Backpacking and Hiking*)

www.insideflyer.com – the latest news from the frequent traveler program that you belong to, includes a run-down of airline, hotel, car-rental, and credit card bonuses, individual program reviews, editorial and proactive leadership on travel-program issues, the Best Bets of special bonuses and awards, and special features such as Mileage Makeover and WiseFlyer

www.joesentme.com – includes a super "Travel Newsstand" section with links to newspaper travel sections and travel magazines around the world, by business-travel guru and all-around nice guy Joe Brancatelli

www.johnnyjet.com – a great collection of resources and information

www.journeywoman.com – a great site for female travelers

www.mobiltravelguide.com – great travel-planning functions as well as helpful ratings of hotels, restaurants, spas, and more

www.momsminivan.com – travel suggestions and games

www.onebag.com – "the art and science of traveling light"

www.vegoutguide.com – great "veg out" guides for travelers, by Margaret Littman (author of *Veg Out Guide to Chicago*)

Travel Supplies

www.aquabells.com/specs.html – Aquabells

www.AquaphorHealing.com – AquaphorHealing

www.claorg.org – Circadian Lighting Association

www.drugstore.com

www.dynamicpainrelief.com – Reflexotherapy Applicator from Dynamic Pain Relief

www.exofficio.com – Buzz Off insect-repellent travel apparel from Ex Officio

www.footsmart.com – FootSmart, compression stockings

www.healthetech.com – Balance Log from HealtheTech

www.magellans.com – Magellan's, America's leading source of travel supplies since 1989 (current catalog available free online or by calling 800-962-4943)

www.mollersupport.com – Moller Back Support System

www.nojetlag.com – NoJetLag

www.protravelgear.com – Pro Travel Gear, dedicated to developing innovative products for the frequent traveler, founded by CEO and veteran pilot David Dillinger

www.purell.com – Purell

www.supportsockshop.com – Support-Sock Shop, compression stockings

www.teplitz.com – *Travel Stress* CD by Jerry V. Teplitz, Ph.D.

www.zicam.com – Zicam

Miscellaneous

www.astanet.com – American Society of Travel Agents

www.countrycallingcodes.com – calling codes from/to any country/city in the world

www.cromwell-intl.com/toilet – "Toilets of the World"

www.dreamofitaly.com – *Dream of Italy*, edited and published by
Kathy McCabe

www.go.hrw.com/atlas/norm_htm/world.htm – an online world atlas

www.indo.com/distance – distances between a huge number of cities
worldwide

www.oanda.com – currency conversion

www.onlinenewspapers.com – newspapers online

www.rv-links.com – a tremendous collection of magazines, books,
and websites dedicated to RV travel

www.seeamerica.org – SeeAmerica, developed by the Travel Industry
Association of America in partnership with more than 2,000 leading
travel industry organizations to promote the United States as the
world's premier tourism destination

www.state.gov – U.S. Department of State

www.timeanddate.com – times (including sunrise and sunset)
around the world

www.tsa.gov – U.S. Transportation Security Administration

www.vortex.bd.psu.edu/~jpp/finitemath/celsfahr.html – Fahrenheit-
Celsius conversions

www.worldtimeserver.com – the time anywhere in the world

TRAVEL MAGAZINES ONLINE

American Way • www.americanwaymag.com

Backpacker • www.backpacker.com

Blue Magazine • www.bluemagazine.com

Cognoscenti • www.cognoscentimag.com

Conde Nast Traveler • www.concierge.com/destination/unitedstates

Dreamscapes • www.dreamscapes.ca

Arthur Frommer's Budget Travel • www.frommers.com

Los Angeles Times Travel Section • www.latimes.com/travel

National Geographic • www.nationalgeographic.com/traveler

RV Journal Magazine • www.newrver.com/rvjournal.html

New York Times Travel Section • www.nytimes.com/travel

Romantic Traveling • www.romantictraveling.com

Spa Magazine • www.spamagazine.com

The TravelInside Info • www.TheTravelInsider.com

Traveler's USA Notebook • www.topquarkia.com

Travel and Leisure Magazine • www.travelandleisure.com

Via • www.viamagazine.com

BOOKS

The Anytime, Anywhere Exercise Book: 300+ Quick and Easy Exercises You Can Do Whenever You Want by Joan Price • www.joanprice.com

The Body Clock Guide to Better Health by Lynne Lamberg • www.bodyclock.com

Caribbean Guide by Janet Groene • www.gordonandjanetgroene.com

Culinary Colorado and *Snowshoeing Colorado* by Claire Walter • www.snowshoeing-colorado.com

The Dog Lover's Companion series by Margaret Littman • www.dogloverscompanion.com

Fitness for Travelers: The Ultimate Workout Guide for the Road by Suzanne Schlosberg • www.suzanneschlosberg.com

Great Eastern RV Trips by Gordon and Janet Groene • www.gordonandjanetgroene.com

Healthy Highways: The Travelers' Guide to Healthy Eating edited by Nikki and David Goldbeck • www.healthyhighways.com

Massachusetts Curiosities: Quirky Characters, Roadside Oddities, and Other Offbeat Stuff by Erik Sherman • www.eriksherman.com

What Are You Hungry For? Women, Food and Spirituality by Lynn Ginsburg and Mary Taylor • www.whatareyouhungryfor.net

Workout on the Go by Karen Bressler • www.amazon.com

The Yankee Chick's Survival Guide to Texas by Sophia Dembling • www.yankeechick.com

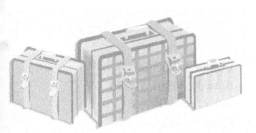

Index

Executive Health Exams
   International, 7
Exercise, 85–94
   clothes, 92
   equipment, 89, 91
   videos and DVDs, 91
   websites, 92–93
Exercises
   isometric, 70, 71
   leg, 78
Exits, 124, 126
Exofficio, 41
Experian, 132
Eyeglasses, 6

F

Fear of flying, 63–66
Feet, 41
Fig Newtons, 108
Film, photographic, 63
Fire ants, 39
Fish, 105
Fit for Business, 92
Flashlights, 124
Flip-flops, 42
Flying anxiety. *See* Fear of flying.
Flying Pilates, 88–89
Flying, 24, 45, 46–48, 81, 110–111
   air pressure, 26–27
   and children, 127
   cabin air, 24–25
   meals, 96–97
   prohibitied items, 61, 63, 120
   seat selection, 46
   security screening, 61–63, 120
   See also Fear of flying.
Focal point, 80
Food

cooked, 105
perishable, 103
raw, 29, 104, 105
safety, 103–105
Four D's, 40
Fragrances, 38
Fribush, Sam, 120
Fruits, 103, 105, 107

G

Ginger root, 34
Goldbeck, David, 97
Goldbeck, Nikki, 97
Golf Bag Shipping, 60
Greco, Megan M., 76
Gridlock, 69–70
Guide to Health Insurance for People with Medicare: Choosing a Medigap Policy, 4
Gum, 27
Gutmann, James, 113
Gyms, 86–90

H

H2 blockers, 29, 31
Hajj, 20
Hand sanitizers, 26
Hand washing, 25, 26
Health advisories, 3
Health
   notebook, 3, 5, 133–162
   records, 7
Hearing loss. *See* Deafness.
Heart attacks, 112
Heartworm, 7
Heatstroke, 41
Heimlich maneuver, 117, 118

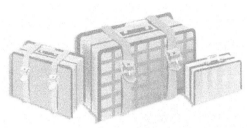

About the Authors

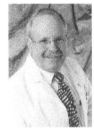

Michael P. Zimring, M.D., is a Board-Certified Internist in private practice with thirty years experience. Dr. Zimring is the Medical Director of the Center for Wilderness and Travel Medicine at Mercy Medical Center in Baltimore, Maryland; the Center (www.travel medicineMD.com) provides pre- and post-travel consultations as well as immunizations in preparation for international travel. He also serves as a Regional Medical Advisor to Medex Assistance (www.medexassist.com), a company that coordinates medical care for international travelers and arranges emergency medical evacuations. An adventure traveler, avid horseman, and naturalist, Dr. Zimring lives in Ellicott City, Maryland with his wife Penny and their two cats, Claws and Rocky.

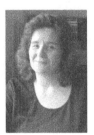

Lisa Iannucci is a twenty-year veteran of magazine and book publishing, having written hundreds of health articles that have appeared in national magazines and newspapers, including the *Los Angeles Times Travel Section, Weight Watchers, Muscle & Fitness, Shape, SkyGuide Go* (American Express), *American Health, USA Weekend, Parenting, New York Magazine,* and more. She is also the author of *The Unofficial Guide to Overcoming Arthritis, The Unofficial Guide to Minding Your Money,* and *Birth Defects.* Ms. Iannucci is also a long-standing member of the American Society of Journalists and Authors and has contributed to *The ASJA Guide to Freelance Writing.*

Visit www.healthytravelbook.com